The Patient's Guide to
AHCC®

Philippa Cheetham, MD

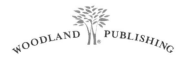

WOODLAND PUBLISHING

Editorial Consultant: Deborah Mitchell

For permissions, ordering information, or bulk quantity discounts, contact:
Woodland Publishing, Salt Lake City, Utah
Visit our website: www.woodlandpublishing.com
Toll-free number: (800) 777-BOOK

The information in this book is for educational purposes only and is not recommended as a means of diagnosing or treating an illness. All matters concerning physical and mental health should be supervised by a health practitioner knowledgeable in treating that particular condition. Neither the publisher nor the author directly or indirectly dispenses medical advice, nor do they prescribe any remedies or assume any responsibility for those who choose to treat themselves.

Cataloging-in-Publication data is available from the Library of Congress

ISBN: 978-1-58054-212-8

Printed in the United States of America

Contents

Introduction

The name may not be engaging or easy to remember, but AHCC® is proving to be an exciting, innovative, effective and memorable nutritional supplement. More precisely, AHCC is not just a supplement; it is a functional food. At its core, AHCC is derived from healing mushrooms. Although mushrooms have long been recognized and honored by various cultures for their medicinal properties and there are numerous mushroom products on the market, AHCC is different from all the rest.

If you are thinking, "Yes, I've heard that line before," or, "Just what we need, another supplement that claims to cure everything," we would have to agree with both of those sentiments. AHCC is different, but does it cure everything? No. Can taking AHCC greatly enhance your health or the health of someone you care about? Most definitely.

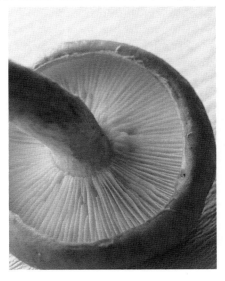

This book shares what experts know about AHCC and individuals have experienced when using this functional food. Scientists have discovered that this potent, versatile gift from nature has impressive immune system enhancing abilities along with anti-inflammatory properties and other healing features. Such characteristics are the core of what makes AHCC such an important product. We discuss these characteristics in greater depth later in the book, but for now let's just say that strengthening and maintaining a strong immune system is instrumental not only in fighting infections such as colds and flu, but also in protecting the body against and treating many serious and chronic diseases such as arthritis, heart disease, autoimmune diseases and cancer because at their core, they may share one thing: they may be controlled by or otherwise intimately associated with, the immune system.

Reducing inflammation is crucial because, although inflammation is the body's natural response to attack, it also is a key element in many serious disorders. Basically, where there's inflammation, there's a problem. Therefore, an effective and safe functional food supplement that can be called upon to help prevent, treat or manage inflammation and other health challenges is highly desirable.

Although AHCC has been studied extensively in both animals and humans for more than 25 years, scientists continue to learn more about it every day, with each new study presenting more insight and knowledge. It is not enough to say, "We have done x number of studies and AHCC is a supplement you should take." We are on a journey of discovery. What has been uncovered thus far has been promising and, in many cases, life changing in small ways as well as big ones. You are invited to join us on this path of opportunity so you can discover how AHCC could make a positive difference in your life.

Chapter 1
AHCC: A Most Remarkable Mushroom

Warning: if you were to look up AHCC in a book on mushrooms or fungi, you would not find it. AHCC is not a genus or species of mushroom but a unique compound extracted from the hybridization of several subspecies of mushrooms. Here is a brief rundown of the birth of AHCC.

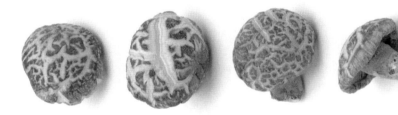

Birth of a Remarkable Mushroom Product

The first component of AHCC is shiitake mushrooms, which have a rich history of healing powers. The next ingredient is several hybrids from the *Basidiomycota* phylum of fungi. Rather than using the "fruiting body"—the familiar cap and stem part of the mushroom that is above ground—AHCC is made using only the mycelia (singular: mycelium), which are the hairlike root structures below the ground. The various mycelia are cultured in a proprietary medium (which possesses antiviral and immune system enhancing qualities of its own) until they form a colony.

The colony is then cultured for an additional 45 to 60 days. The resulting product undergoes a series of patented steps that involve cultivation, decomposition by enzymes, sterilization, concentration and freeze-drying, all developed at the University of Tokyo Faculty of Pharmaceutical Sciences by Dr. Toshihiko Okamoto, along with researchers at Amino Up Chemical Co., Ltd. in Japan. The end result of this carefully computer-monitored manufacturing process is the functional food supplement AHCC, a product with impressive and growing evidence of effectiveness and an impeccable safety profile (see more on safety on page 63).

One special part of the manufacturing process occurs when the enzymes break down the nutrients in the mycelia into a form that is better absorbed by the body. This process results in AHCC having a much lower molecular weight (5,000 daltons) when compared with other mushroom extracts, which average 100,000 daltons or higher. This low molecular weight is a unique feature of AHCC. A low molecular weight allows the body to utilize the compounds in AHCC in an optimal manner. In particular, the immune system's white blood cells have easy access to AHCC's constituents so they can use them to strengthen the body's defenses and fight tumors. So what are those nutrients?

AHCC: Much More Than a Fungus

The chemical composition of AHCC includes: carbohydrates (44 percent), fats (37.3 percent), proteins (7.2 percent), vitamins B_1, B_2 and B_3 (niacin) (0.3 percent each), fiber, minerals (4.5 percent each, sodium and potassium) and water (1.3 percent). (Amounts are approximate.) Most of the carbohydrates are polysaccharides, complex carbohydrates formed by the bonding of various monosaccharides, which include sugars such as glucose and fructose. The "secret" of AHCC's activity in the body lies in its unique composition that includes highly bioactive alpha-glucans and other compounds such as axoglucans™ fractions.

One such fraction called "Active Hexose Correlated Compound" is a combination of two compounds: glucosyl-isomaltol and maltosyl-isomaltol. Being a subject of one of the original patents on AHCC, it initially received a lot of attention from researchers and started being cited in various published studies. However, subsequent research showed that active hexose correlated compound is present in very low quantities and is not bioactive. Therefore, this fraction is not believed to contribute to the efficacy of AHCC.

Excuse us if we get a bit technical here, but an explanation of

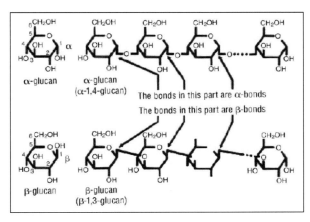

alpha-glucans can help you better understand why AHCC is much more than a fungus. First of all, polysaccharides are the active compounds in many healing foods and supplements made from mushrooms and plants. The primary polysaccharides in other mushroom-based health foods are beta-glucans. The words "alpha" and "beta" refer to the types of bonds each glucan has with sugar (glucose) molecules.

The main polysaccharides in AHCC are acylated alpha-glucan (specifically, alpha-1,4-glucan). The presence of acylated alpha-glucan makes AHCC unique and especially effective. The word "acylated" means adding an acyl group (CH3CO-) to glucan. This occurs during the long culturing process that is part of the manufacturing of AHCC. Acylated alpha-glucan has a molecular weight of 5,000 daltons while beta-glucans are much higher and thus more difficult for the body to digest and absorb.

The acylated alpha-glucans, however, are the stars and the unique component of AHCC. They directly impact the immune system after they are digested and absorbed by the body. Various scientists have explored the activities and functions of alpha-glucans versus beta-glucans, including a team at the Cancer Research Unit of the Pathology Division of the Department of Medicine, Hokkaido University in Sapporo, Japan. The researchers divided each component of AHCC into those with high molecular weight and low molecular weight (e.g., alpha-glucans) and studied their effect on cancer-bearing mice.

When the scientists examined the cancer cells in mice that received AHCC components of high molecular weight versus those of low molecular weight, they noted that certain immune system cells called interleukin-12 and tumor necrosis factor-alpha (beneficial immune cells that we discuss in detail in the next chapter) were induced. However, induction of interleukin-12 was strongest when low molecular weight components were given. Experts also know that the low molecular weight polysaccharides of AHCC are mainly effective in improving the production abilities of immune system elements that have potent immune-stimulating actions. In other words, high-molecular weight beta-glucans are not nearly as effective as low-molecular weight alpha-glucans.

"Radical" Ideas about Infections and Disease

What is a disease? If your doctor gives you a diagnosis of heart disease, you automatically assume you have a heart problem and your doctor treats your heart. Similarly, if you have benign prostatic hyperplasia, a disease characterized by an enlarged prostate gland, you have a problem with that specific gland and you are given a treatment plan for your prostate. This makes sense, right? Yes and not necessarily.

Recently, experts within the conventional medical arena have been exploring the idea that some health conditions affect the entire body, even though they may appear to involve only the heart, lungs, prostate or other organ or body part. This is a more holistic and encompassing perspective of disease and health and introduces the idea that since the immune system is present throughout and affects the entire body and thus can impact the activity of every organ and organ system, it makes sense to strengthen the immune system in order to fight, prevent and/or treat a wide variety of health problems.

In a study published in 2000 in *Biotherapy*, Katsuaki Uno, MD, a cancer researcher and oncologist who uses AHCC for his cancer patients, pointed out that in order for cancer cells to develop into a tumor, they require a certain environment or "diseased condition," one that is the result of a deterioration of the immune system. He has stated that "cancer is an abnormality of immunity that brings about the onset of diseases—it's a disease of immunity."

This may be a radical idea for some people, but it is gaining a lot of attention and supporting evidence. In the same article, Uno also explained that "many specialists have come to realize that abnormalities of immunity play a fundamental role in the deterioration of 'diseases of lifestyle,' conditions in which the system is overtaxed, such as arteriosclerosis and high blood pressure, into the onset of cerebral vascular disease, cardiovascular disease, diabetes and other conditions."

In other words, if your immune system has been weakened and is struggling for any number of reasons ranging from stress to poor nutrition to exposure to environmental toxins, it provides a fertile environment for disease to take hold. And we are not talking about just an invasion of disease-causing bacteria and other microorganisms that can result in the common cold or flu or hepatitis, but chronic diseases not typically associated with infections, such as heart disease, diabetes and arthritis.

So here is the other part of the "radical" idea: Scientists have found a possible connection between microorganisms and chronic diseases not previously believed to be caused by infections. In fact, researchers have made a connection between microorganisms and arteriosclerosis, rheumatoid arthritis, polycystic ovary disease, some forms of cancer, multiple sclerosis, duodenal ulcers, diabetes, heart disease, Alzheimer's disease, various psychiatric disorders and others.

Therefore, the concept of strengthening and supporting the immune system with a functional food supplement like AHCC is feasible because (as you will learn later in this book) research strongly indicates that AHCC has the ability to positively strengthen, enhance or otherwise improve the immune system's response to elements that threaten to harm the body. Immune system strength is the key and gateway to physical and mental health.

Now, before we explore the immune system in detail and the intimate relationship between AHCC and components of the immune system, let's look at some special features of AHCC.

AHCC as Immunomodulator

An immunomodulator is a substance that changes, suppresses or strengthens the immune system. Chemical examples include methotrexate and azathioprine, drugs that are often used to treat the immune response in people who have various cancers, psoriasis or rheumatoid arthritis. Chemical immunomodulators, however, are a double-edged sword. Methotrexate can slow the growth of cancer cells and skin cells, as well as suppress the immune system in rheumatoid arthritis patients, but it can also damage bone marrow and reduce the number of red blood cells, along with damaging the liver.

AHCC presents a broader effect than chemical immunomodulators in that it has a normalizing function. That is, it can stimulate the immune system when immune response is inhibited, but it can also calm excessive immune reactions. An example of this dual ability can be seen in how AHCC affects cancer cells.

As you will learn on page 17 where the immune system is discussed in detail, AHCC can stimulate production of a substance called tumor necrosis factor alpha (TNF-a). This substance promotes the breakdown of tumors, which makes it a good candidate for cancer treatment. TNF-a also has a pro-inflammatory effect, which is a problem in people who have arthritis. The good news is that AHCC has shown that it can also stimulate the reduction of TNF-a in people who have rheumatoid arthritis. This is an example of AHCC's normalizing function and it appears to be the result of AHCC's ability to strengthen the function of the immune system in the area of the body where it is most needed.

AHCC and Inflammation

Inflammation is a reaction of the immune system in response to trauma, infection or irritation. Characteristic responses include a rush of white blood cells to the area involved, along with heat, swelling, pain and dysfunction of the tissues or organs affected. Inflammation stimulates the immune system and is a critical first step in the process of fighting an infection and healing damaged cells and tissues. However, when inflammation is chronic, which means the immune system is always in alert mode, it can lead to chronic conditions.

In recent years, scientists have discovered that inflammation plays a major role in a great number of chronic diseases. Included are allergic disorders, such as allergic asthma, atopic dermatitis and pollen allergies; autoimmune disorders such as rheumatoid arthritis, lupus and ulcerative colitis; and a number of other conditions you may not associate with inflammation, such as Alzheimer's disease, cancer, diabetes, heart disease, irritable bowel syndrome (IBS), obesity, Parkinson's disease and more. This discovery has given scientists and clinicians a better understanding of these conditions as well as new ways to approach treatment. AHCC may be a part of one of those treatments approaches.

AHCC has anti-inflammatory properties, which makes it a potential candidate for addressing diseases characterized by inflammation. One very effective way to monitor the level of inflammation in the body is to measure the amount of a protein in the bloodstream called C-reactive protein or CRP. When levels of CRP are high, this signals the presence of infections, certain cancers, inflammatory bowel disease, pancreatitis, cardiovascular disease and other inflammatory conditions. Research has also shown that AHCC may reduce inflammation and high levels of CRP.

AHCC may also increase levels of leptin, a hormone with anti-inflammatory properties. Dr. Satoru Yui of Teikyo University Department of Pharmacology in Tokyo, Japan, reports that AHCC is capable of increasing levels of this anti-inflammatory agent. Leptin is also involved in weight control because it is instrumental in the metabolism of fat and in regulating appetite. This suggests AHCC could be helpful in controlling weight.

Current conventional treatments for inflammation typically include medications such as steroids and nonsteroidal anti-inflammatory drugs (NSAIDs), which are associated with significant side effects, including gastrointestinal bleeding and nausea. Some NSAIDs may damage the immune system. AHCC could provide a safe, effective alternative. AHCC could also be used along with these drugs to enhance healing as well as have a positive impact on the underlying cause of the disease.

How AHCC is Studied

One of the challenges scientists face when researching ways to treat infectious diseases is that there are no ethical, reliable or practical means to evaluate the human response to infectious agents. However, what researchers can and do perform are studies using animal models, which allow them to demonstrate the efficacy of AHCC. They also conduct human clinical trials, which allow them to show AHCC's ability to act on the many components of the immune system.

That is why you will notice that some of the studies discussed throughout this book have been done on mice. Mice are highly homologous, or structurally similar, to humans and the strains of mice used in biomedical research have been genetically designed so scientists can accurately reproduce the same strains again and again. This helps ensure investigators are comparing "apples with apples," so to speak, when conducting research.

Research mice have critical characteristics that make them ideal for drug testing as well as for research of a range of human diseases and conditions. Scientists have developed strains of inbred mice to produce test mice with Alzheimer's disease, arthritis, lupus, ulcers, inflammatory bowel disease, diabetes, obesity and a wide range of cancers, among other conditions.

Therefore, a combination of animal models, human clinical studies and human case reports are the proving grounds for AHCC, and these are the grounds we will explore throughout this book.

Wrap-Up

AHCC is a remarkable mushroom product, displaying anti-inflammatory, immune system enhancing, immunomodulatory and antioxidant properties. Such characteristics make AHCC a likely candidate for a broad spectrum of health issues ranging from the common cold to cancer. Why? Because most of the ailments and diseases that affect people are intimately associated with the immune system. If you boost and strengthen immune functioning and immune response, then you can gain an upper hand in fighting these illnesses and diseases. And that's where AHCC enters the picture. The relationship between AHCC and the immune system is a complex and intimate one and one that is explored in the next section.

Chapter 2
Introducing Your Immune System

The immune system is something people tend to take for granted until they need it. The truth is, however, that you always need it, even when you're feeling completely healthy. Your immune system is constantly "on," monitoring your body for any chink in the armor: the presence of abnormal cells, renegade cell growth and antigens (unwelcome bacteria, viruses, fungi, parasites, toxins and other organisms that could trigger a health problem). However, the individual components of your immune system need to be "on" as well, primed to act when called upon. If one or more of those components are inadequate, then overall health can suffer.

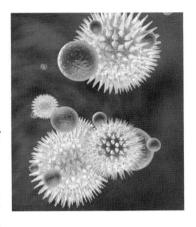

Considering the critical role the immune system plays in your health, it is worth taking some time to understand it better. Knowing how your immune system functions—and especially the ways AHCC interacts with it—can help you better appreciate how AHCC can improve your health.

The immune system is the body's defense against infectious organisms and other unwelcome substances. Through a series of steps called the immune response, the immune system identifies, targets and attacks the bacteria, viruses and other antigens that can cause disease.

Components of the Immune System

The immune system is a complex network that involves many different cells, tissues and organs that have varying and often interconnected roles. (See list starting on page 19). The main cells involved in immune system functioning are white blood cells or leukocytes, of which there are two basic types: macrophages, which "eat up" abnormal cells and invading organisms; and lymphocytes, which destroy foreign substances, produce chemicals that act as messengers, and allow the body to remember and recognize previous invaders so the body can destroy them.

The key transportation apparatus for the immune system is the lymphatic system, which is a combination of organs, nodes and ducts that transport a watery clear fluid called lymph, or lymphatic fluid, throughout the body. The lymphatic fluid performs several critical functions: it delivers nutrients and chemical messengers to the body's cells and it interacts with the blood circulatory system to carry away waste materials from the cells.

The immune system also includes the spleen, tonsils, thymus gland, adenoids and sections of the small intestine, all of which are composed of lymphoid tissue, where lymphocytes are formed. Other important players in the immune system are bone marrow and mucous membranes, which are found throughout the body as well. In fact, lymphatic tissue is found in every part of the body except the central nervous system. The heart, lungs, intestinal tract, liver and skin also contain lymphatic tissue and thus are intimately connected to the immune system. When we say that AHCC has an

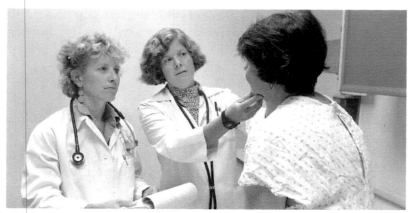

Image courtesy of Seattle Municipal Archives via Flickr® creative commons

impact on the entire immune system, it follows that it has an impact on nearly all parts of the body.

Lymphocytes start out their lives in the bone marrow and either stay there and mature into B lymphocytes (B cells) or they migrate to the thymus gland, where they turn into T lymphocytes (T cells). The T cells and B cells have a close working relationship: B cells seek out invading organisms and send in forces to attack them, while T cells destroy the invaders once they have been identified.

Macrophages also arise from the bone marrow. These white blood cells ingest bacteria and other harmful organisms in a process called phagocytosis. Macrophages get some assistance from other white blood cells called neutrophils.

Here is a brief review of some of the players involved in immune function. Many of these factors work together in its effort to support and maintain an optimally functioning immune system. We will refer to these various immune components a great deal throughout the book.

- **Antigens:** Antigens are substances—bacteria, viruses, toxins, foreign blood cells—that when introduced into the body stimulate the production of an antibody, which can then neutralize the antigens.
- **T lymphocytes (T cells):** A type of white blood cell involved in various immune functions. There are several subtypes of T cells, including helper T cells, suppressor T cells and cytotoxic T cells.
  - **Helper T** cells do not kill cancer cells or germs directly, but they release substances that help B cells and killer T cells work better. There are also three types of helper T cells, two of which we are concerned with: helper T1 (Th1), which are involved in cell-mediated immunity; and helper T2 (Th2), which are involved in humoral immunity
  - **Suppressor T cells** help make sure the immune system does not overreact and attack other healthy parts of the body
  - **Cytotoxic T cells (killer T cells)** release substances that kill abnormal cells and invading organisms in the body
- **B lymphocytes (B cells):** B cells are produced in the bone marrow and mature into plasma cells. They are responsible for the production of antibodies, which are key in the fight against bacterial infections.

- **Dendritic cells (DCs):** White blood cells that process antigens (foreign materials) and present them to B and T cells. Thus DCs are the "delivery boys" of the immune system: although B cells and T cells are the mediators of immunity, their function is under the control of DCs. This activity is especially important with respect to AHCC, because AHCC stimulates an increase in the number of DCs.

- **Macrophages:** Macrophages are white blood cells that consume abnormal cells and invading organisms.

- **Natural killer cells (NK):** A type of lymphocyte that performs a critical job in the immune system: NK cells can detect and destroy tumor cells and microbes before they reproduce, which can protect you from chronic, degenerative diseases. NK cells work by latching onto a cancer cell or microbe and injecting a granule into its victim, which causes the cell or microbe to die. The activity of NK cells is an indication of the strength of the immune system and is also used to determine the prognosis of cancer and AIDS patients. When NK activity declines to zero, death occurs.

- **Lymphokine activated killer cells (LAK):** A type of white blood cell that has been stimulated to destroy tumor cells.

- **Neutrophils:** The most common type of white blood cell and the type most responsible for immune response. Neutrophils are present in the bloodstream until they are called to action at an infection site. After they ingest other cells, they die.

- **CD4:** These glycoproteins are found on the surface of T helper cells, macrophages and dendritic cells. These "helper" cells initiate the body's response to outside invaders such as bacteria and viruses.

- **CD8:** These glycoproteins are mostly found on the surface of cytotoxic T cells, but also on NK cells and dendritic cells. They are involved in destroying cells that are infected with foreign microorganisms.

- **CD4/CD8 ratio:** Clinicians can use this ratio to determine how strong the immune system is and to help predict the risk of complications.

- **Cytokines:** Chemicals that act as messengers between cells to direct and enhance immune response. There are several types of cytokines:
  - **Interferon** protects cells from viruses, destroys cancer tumors and stimulates NK cells and macrophages
  - **Interleukin-2 (IL-2)** stimulates the growth and activity of T cells
  - **Interleukin-12 (IL-12)** stimulates NK cells and strengthens cellular immunity
  - **Transforming growth factor beta (TGF-b)** is a protein that controls proliferation, cellular differentiation and other cell functions. It has an important role in immunity and cancer, as cancerous cells increase their production of TGF-b
  - **Tumor necrosis factor (TNF)** is a cytokine that is involved in the inflammatory process and that is capable of killing tumor cells

- **Lymph nodes:** Bean-shaped structures where lymphocytes often are first exposed to bacteria, viruses and other antigens, which stimulates the lymphocytes to perform their functions. Lymph nodes, which form in clusters throughout the immune system, can become enlarged due to infection or a tumor.

- **Spleen:** An organ that processes lymphocytes that enter it from incoming blood.

- **Tonsils and adenoids:** Structures that are composed of tissues similar to those in the lymph nodes. Together the tonsils and adenoids are part of a ring that encircles the back of the throat and they are thought to help the body fight invading microorganisms.

Immune System: A Duet

The immune system has two main divisions, humoral immunity and cellular (cell mediated) immunity and these two divisions complement or play off of each other.

Humoral immunity is the part of immunity that is mediated by the secretion of antibodies produced by B lymphocytes and other processes that facilitate them, such as Th2 activation and the production of cytokines. These antibodies attach themselves to antigens, which marks them for destruction. Humoral immunity gets its name from the word "humours," a word that comes from ancient times and refers to substances that ancient physicians thought were found in bodily fluids.

Cell-mediated immunity is an immune response that involves activation of various immune components, such as macrophages, natural killer cells, cytotoxic T lymphocytes and various cytokines, all in response to invasion by antigens. In cell-mediated immunity, these and other immune cells release toxins to kill bacteria, viruses and other antigens or they attack the unwelcome organisms directly to kill them.

AHCC and Your Immune System

Taoist philosopher Lao Tzu said, "Health is the greatest possession." To possess health, you need a strong immune system: If you keep your immune system operating at an optimal level, then you greatly increase your chances of avoiding and preventing infections, disease and other health problems. In today's world, it can be difficult at times to protect your immune system from the assaults of microorganisms, stress, poor nutrition, lack of sleep, environmental toxins, medications and other threats. Although the immune system is extremely resilient, it also takes work on your part to keep it operating optimally.

If your overall health is good and you don't have any pressing health problems, then you are ahead of the game. However, that does not mean you should let your guard down. "Health is not valued till sickness comes" is a grim reminder from 17th century British writer Thomas Fuller. If you already have one or more health conditions that are challenging you, supporting and protecting your immune system is even more critical.

AHCC is a functional food supplement that can help protect your immune system both when it is functioning well and when it is not. That is, it can protect you from getting sick as well as tackle the factors that cause you to be sick.

How AHCC Strengthens the Immune System

Numerous studies show that AHCC has the ability to promote and stimulate significant changes in the immune system. We explore the activities and functions of AHCC in more detail in subsequent sections when we talk about how AHCC works with infections, cancer, gastrointestinal disorders, your liver, diabetes and your heart. For now, here is a brief look at what research has shown about the impact AHCC has on some of the components of the immune system we have already mentioned.

- **Macrophages:** AHCC can significantly increase the number of macrophages, which in turn improves the ability of the immune system to function optimally. Because cellular immunity is initiated when macrophages and neutrophils are activated, AHCC can play a major role in jump-starting this process, especially in individuals with a compromised immune system. The activity of macrophages was demonstrated in a mouse model of breast cancer. Breast cancer was transplanted into two groups of mice, with one group also receiving an injection of AHCC. After one month, the tumor had shrunk in size by 60 percent in the AHCC-treated mice compared with the untreated mice. The presence of tumor necrosis factor-alpha (TNF-a) was confirmed in the AHCC-treated mice. TNF-a is mainly produced by macrophages, thus it was assumed that the cancer cells were acted on by a combination of factors: they were attacked by the macrophages and subsequently destroyed by the TNF-a.

- **Cytokines:** Both animal and human studies show that AHCC can increase the levels of cytokines, including TNF, interferon-gamma and the interleukins 1 and 12 (IL-1, IL-12). In addition, AHCC can inhibit the activity of cytokines that suppress the immune system, such as TGF-b. In a study conducted by Dr. Katsuaki Uno of Comfort Hospital, 38 people with stage IV cancer were given six grams daily of AHCC. After four months of treatment, the levels of IL-12 approached the levels seen in healthy individuals in 90 percent of the patients, and a similar increase was seen in interferon-gamma levels, with a corresponding increase in the activity of cytotoxic T cells as these latter levels rose.

- **Natural killer cells:** Studies in people with cancer show that AHCC can elevate the activity level of NK cells by 200 to 300 percent. This ability to increase NK activity is critically important, because NK cells detect and fight abnormal cells, including cancer cells. The activity of NK cells also appears to have an additive effect on chemotherapy: patients undergoing chemotherapy have demonstrated an enhanced response to treatment when they take AHCC.

- **Dendritic cells: (DCs):** A study published in *Nutrition and Cancer* reports that healthy individuals who took AHCC daily for one month had a significant increase in their DC levels compared with those who took a placebo.
- **T cells:** Numerous studies, including several conducted at Yale School of Medicine, have shown that AHCC increases the number and effectiveness of T cells as much as 200 percent.
- **T helper (Th) cells:** AHCC can improve the balance between Th1 and Th2 cells, which are involved in activating and directing other immune system cell functions, including activation and growth of cytotoxic lymphocytes and maximizing the activities of macrophages.

AHCC and Older Adults

Although AHCC can benefit immune function for people of all ages, we want to make a special mention here of how the supplement can benefit older adults, with examples from two studies. The gradual deterioration of the immune system that occurs with advancing age is called "immunosenescence." This type of immunodeficiency causes the elderly to be more susceptible to infectious conditions ranging from the flu and the common cold to pneumonia, cancer and other serious conditions.

In one study, AHCC was shown to stimulate T cell function in adults aged 50 years and older. At Yale School of Medicine, Zhinan Yin, MD, a rheumatologist, and his colleagues evaluated the impact of AHCC on a group of 30 healthy adults. Each study participant had his or her cytokine production measured by the CD4+ and CD8+ cells before taking AHCC, after 30 days on AHCC, after 60 days and again 30 days after they stopped treatment. (Remember, the CD4/CD8 ratio tells clinicians how strong the immune system is.)

The researchers observed significant and consistent increases in the CD4+ cells' production of both interferon-gamma and TNF-a, two key cytokines in the body's natural defenses against cancer-causing cells, within four weeks of AHCC supplementation. The increased production remained for the entire treatment period. At 30 days post-treatment, cytokine production by CD4+ had declined.

AHCC had a different effect on CD8+ cells. Although AHCC did not initiate much in the way of increased cytokine production after 30 and 60 days of supplementation, the researchers saw a significant increase in both cytokines 30 days after treatment stopped. These findings suggest that AHCC is effective both during treatment and after people stop taking it. Yin's study was also the first to show that AHCC could be beneficial in relieving immunosenescence and thus could prove to be helpful in preventing the development of some conditions that affect older adults.

The second study we want to mention was a double-blind, randomized trial that included 21 healthy adults with an average age of 60. Each subject received a placebo or three grams of AHCC daily for four weeks. The researchers collected blood samples both at the start of the study and at four weeks. The blood samples showed that subjects who took AHCC had significantly higher levels of total DCs and showed increased function of DCs compared to baseline and to controls. These findings are significant because DCs are, in the words of the study's lead author, Naoyoshi Terakawa, MD, of Kansai Medical University, "critical for maintaining a healthy and balanced immune system."

Wrap-Up

The immune system is a complex network of many different cells, tissues and organs designed to keep harmful invaders out or, when they do infiltrate, to hunt down, attack and destroy them. AHCC supports, strengthens and enhances immune system components so they can better perform the job they were designed to do.

Chapter 3
Colds, Flu and Other Infections

You would be hard-pressed to find someone who has not experienced an infectious disease. Have you had a cold recently? Then you had an infectious disease. The flu? Ditto. Not to mention pneumonia, urinary tract infections, fungal infections and more. If you have a loved one who is a resident in a nursing home or other medical facility, you may worry about an outbreak of MRSA (methicillin-resistant *Staphylococcus aureus*) or other antibiotic-resistant infections. Cases of West Nile virus crop up each year in nearly every state in the nation and the threat of avian (bird) flu still lingers. One of the best ways to protect yourself and your family against these and other infectious diseases is by strengthening your immune system with AHCC.

Fighting Infections

The standard approach to killing germs in the home and other environments, as well as in our bodies, has been "overkill"—overuse of antibacterial soaps, sprays and other antibacterial products and the over-prescribing of antibiotics. This zealous approach to fighting germs and preventing infections has, unfortunately, largely backfired because we now have to fight "superbugs"—bacteria that have become resistant to the antibiotics that were developed to attack and destroy them.

Given the ineffectiveness of antibiotics, not to mention the fact that they are associated with side effects and can make you susceptible to even more infections, many people are turning to natural alternatives. Among the more common nutritional and herbal supplements people take to enhance their immune systems in an attempt to ward off or treat infections are vitamin C, echinacea, garlic and ginseng, among others (see page 64). Generally, these supplements have not been rigorously studied in response to infectious diseases and results of the studies that have been done have provided mixed and often conflicting findings.

AHCC has been studied extensively and offers a way to prevent and treat infections from the front line: building up, strengthening and supporting the immune system by activating specific immune cells such as NK cells, among others, and enhancing their activities. Let's take a look at the more common infections shown to respond to AHCC and the studies that support the use of AHCC in preventing and fighting infectious diseases.

Cold and Flu

At the top of the infectious disease list are the common cold and the flu. The National Institute of Allergy and Infectious Diseases notes that people in the United States suffer one billion colds per year, according to some estimates. Children are usually the hardest hit, as they average six to 10 colds 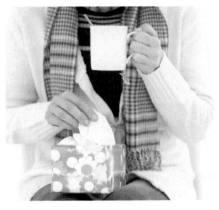 per year while adults usually get two to four, with people older than 60 experiencing the fewest colds (but not the least number of other infections, which we will talk about later). However, while older adults may contract fewer colds, they often have a longer and more difficult time recovering from them.

According to the Centers for Disease Control and Prevention (CDC), up to 20 percent of Americans get the flu each year. While the flu certainly disrupts the lives of millions of people by making them feel too ill to go to work or school, for some people it is much more serious. The CDC reports that more than 200,000 people are hospitalized because of flu each year and about 36,000 die. With the appearance of bird (avian) flu and swine flu (H1N1) in recent years, the word "flu" has taken on new, more dire meaning for many people, especially the very young, pregnant women, the elderly and anyone whose immune system is already compromised.

The Studies

The need for a reliable, potent immune system enhancer to help ward off the common cold and flu is great. Studies showing the efficacy of AHCC have been and continue to be conducted. One of the first studies in this arena was done at Drexel University in Philadelphia and reported in the *Journal of Nutrition* in 2006. Researchers used two groups of mice: one group was infected with influenza A (H1N1) flu only (control group) and the other group was administered AHCC (one g/kg/body weight per day) for one week before they were infected with the flu and throughout the course of infection.

The researchers found that the AHCC-treated mice had increased survival, decreased severity of symptoms and a shorter recovery after they were infected than did the control mice. Specifically, use of AHCC reduced the death rate from 25 percent to five percent.

In addition, the investigators found that use of AHCC increased the activity of NK cells in the lungs one day after infection and in the spleen two days after infection. Such rapid and increased activity means AHCC facilitated the clearance of the virus from the body. The AHCC-treated mice also maintained their body weight during the infection when compared with controls, which is an indication the treated mice experienced less severe disease. The study's authors concluded that use of a dietary bioactive substance such as AHCC "may be one avenue for improving the immune response to primary flu infection."

In two other studies, researchers looked at the effectiveness of AHCC in mice that were infected with the H5N1 avian influenza virus, also known as the bird flu. In one study, published in the *Japanese Journal of Complementary and Alternative Medicine*, control mice were infected with the virus, while another group of mice was given AHCC daily for seven days before they were infected with 100 times the 50 percent lethal dose of H5N1 flu virus. All the control mice died by day 11 after they were infected, while 30 percent of the AHCC-treated mice were still alive 28 days post-infection.

In the second study, the scientists followed the same protocol, but this time they compared the effects of AHCC alone to H5N1 vaccination alone, as well as the combination of AHCC and the flu vaccine given together. In the mice that received the H5N1 vaccination only, approximately 80 percent survived the infection. However, 100 percent of the mice that received both the vaccination and AHCC survived.

When the results of these two studies of bird flu are considered together, we find that AHCC provides some protection against this virus, yet combining AHCC with the vaccine appears to be more effective.

The idea of combining AHCC with a flu vaccine was then tested in a small double-blind, placebo-controlled human trial. The 29 people in the study all received the flu vaccination and then for two weeks after the vaccination, half took 3,000 mg AHCC daily while the other half took a placebo. Blood samples were taken from all participants on the day of vaccination and again two weeks later.

The post-vaccination blood samples of the people who took AHCC showed elevated levels of immune cells, including T cells (especially cytotoxic cells) and a type of NK cells that produce cytokines in response to the flu vaccine. This enhanced response was most evident in adults older than 60, who are at greater risk of complications due to flu. The results of this study led the authors to note, "This suggests that short-term AHCC supplementation may be a good therapeutic intervention to sustain or increase, the immune response to influenza vaccination in healthy subjects."

Although no studies have yet been conducted to explore the impact of AHCC on the common cold, the ability of AHCC to promote the activity of NK cells shortly after infection, as demonstrated in the flu research, suggests it will prove beneficial. There is also convincing evidence suggested by the results of yet more studies of the activity of AHCC against other infectious diseases, as shown on pages 29–34.

West Nile Virus

Despite its name, the West Nile virus can affect people who do not live anywhere near the Nile. Basically, if there are mosquitoes where you live, there is a chance you could contract West Nile virus. In 2010, the CDC noted that approximately 1,000 cases of the virus had been reported to the agency, with 41 deaths. The three states reporting more than 100 cases each were Arizona, California and New York.

About one in 150 people who are infected with West Nile virus develop severe illness, with symptoms that include high fever, headache, stupor, disorientation, coma, tremors, convulsions, numbness and paralysis. Symptoms may last a few weeks and the neurological impact may be permanent. Up to 20 percent of infected individuals have milder symptoms—fever, headache, body aches, nausea, vomiting and swollen glands or rash. These symptoms usually last for a few days, but even healthy people can be ill for several weeks. About 80 percent of people who are infected with West Nile virus don't display any symptoms.

Thus far, there are no vaccines or treatments to prevent or treat this virus. AHCC, however, has shown promise in the fight against this sometimes fatal disease.

For example, at Colorado State University, a team of scientists evaluated the ability of AHCC to enhance resistance when exposed to West Nile virus. They used a mouse model, with one group of mice administered 600 mg/kg of AHCC every other day for one week before they were infected with a lethal dose of West Nile virus. The mice were given AHCC on days one and three after they were infected as well. Mice in the control group received a placebo and the deadly dose.

One month later, an analysis of the animals' blood showed that AHCC had increased the production of antibodies for West Nile virus in the treated mice. Overall, mice treated with AHCC had 19 percent less viral load than the control mice and were also twice as likely to have survived the lethal dose: 54 percent of treated mice were still alive compared with only 21 percent of the control mice. The authors, who published their work in the *Journal of Nutrition*, reported that "dietary supplementation with AHCC may be potentially immunotherapeutic for WNV-susceptible populations."

AHCC and "Superbug" Bacterial Infections

Although the use of antibiotics can be beneficial in some cases, overuse of these drugs has resulted in the emergence of antibiotic-resistant strains of bacteria or "superbugs." This means that when clinicians are presented with patients who have a bacterial infection caused by microorganisms known to be resistant to antibiotics that were once effective, they and their patients are faced with a treatment challenge that can all too often result in serious complications or even death.

Pseudomonas aeruginosa infections, for example, which frequently occur in people who have a compromised immune system, cause death in half of those who develop this opportunistic infection. (An opportunistic infection is one that is caused by microorganisms that usually do not cause illness but do when the individual's immune system has been compromised and thus cannot fight off the infection.)

Along with *P. aeruginosa*, there are two other opportunistic infections that are important to understand and against which AHCC has been shown to be effective, MRSA and *Klebsiella pneumonia*.

Pseudomonas aeruginosa Infections

Pseudomonas aeruginosa is an opportunistic infection that often affects people who have compromised immune systems and rarely affects uncompromised tissues. However, *P. aeruginosa* is relentless when it does infect tissues, causing urinary tract infections, respiratory tract infections, dermatitis, ear infections, endocarditis, meningitis, brain abscesses, soft tissue infections, bone and joint infections, gastrointestinal infections, bacteremia and various other systemic infections. Among people at high risk for *P. aeruginosa* infections are individuals who have AIDS, cancer, severe burns or cystic fibrosis. Among patients who are hospitalized with these conditions, the fatality rate is about 50 percent.

Pseudomonas has a reputation for being resistant to antibiotics. Among the few that are effective against the bacteria are fluoroquinolones, gentamicin and imipenem, yet they are not able to kill all strains. Perhaps the population hit the hardest with *P. aeruginosa* infections are cystic fibrosis patients, because nearly all of them eventually contract a strain that is so resistant to antibiotics that they cannot be treated successfully.

AHCC has proven effective against *P. aeruginosa* in a study conducted at Teikyo University School of Medicine in Japan. Researchers evaluated the effect of different doses of AHCC given by injection and orally to immune-compromised mice and found that the mushroom compound protected the mice from lethal infection with *P. aeruginosa*.

Specifically, the mice that received 500 mg/kg of AHCC by injection survived an average of 14 days after they were infected with *P. aeruginosa* compared with only three days among the control (untreated) mice. Oral AHCC provided a similar result, with six of the eight mice treated with 1,000 mg/kg of AHCC surviving 14 days compared with only three days among the control mice.

MRSA

Another infection that has many people concerned is MRSA. This is a type of staph bacterial infection that is resistant to certain antibiotics called beta-lactams, which include methicillin, oxacillin, penicillin and amoxicillin. Among the general population, most MRSA infections affect the skin. In healthcare settings such as nursing homes and hospitals, however, the infections are typically more severe or potentially life-threatening. The CDC reports that in 2005, about 94,360 people developed MRSA and that more than 18,000 people died. The effectiveness of AHCC was tested in mice that were given both oral and injectable doses of the compound. Mice that were treated with AHCC survived significantly longer after receiving a lethal dose of MRSA than did mice that received a placebo.

Klebsiella pneumonia Infections

Klebsiella pneumonia is among the most common gram-negative bacteria healthcare providers encounter around the world. It is often found in hospitals, where it usually causes urinary tract infections, nosocomial pneumonia (pneumonia that develops as a result of treatment in a hospital or other healthcare setting) and intra-abdominal infections. People most at risk for developing a *K. pneumonia* infection include anyone who is using a ventilator or who has an intravenous catheter or patients who are on a prolonged course of antibiotics. Healthy individuals rarely get *Klebsiella* infections.

Several studies have looked at the impact of AHCC on resistance to infection with *K. pneumonia* and the results have been promising. In one, published in the *Journal of Applied Physiology*, investigators chose a mouse model that is often used for spaceflight conditions (e.g., suspension) because spaceflight conditions impair immune function. The scientists administered AHCC to the mice one week before they were infected with *K. pneumonia* and were suspended and throughout the 10-day suspension period as well. Mice that received AHCC had decreased mortality, longer survival and an increased ability to clear the deadly bacteria from their bodies than did control mice that did not receive AHCC.

Another study evaluated how effective AHCC may be in

preventing surgical wound infections caused by *K. pneumonia* in a mouse model. The 28 treated mice in the study were administered an oral dose of AHCC daily for eight days before and during the time they were infected with *K. pneumonia*. A control group of 28 mice received a placebo and were also infected with the bacteria. The AHCC-treated mice survived longer than the control mice: 15 percent of control and 55 percent of treated mice were alive after 15 days. The AHCC-treated mice also cleared the infection much more effectively than did the control mice. This suggests to scientists that AHCC

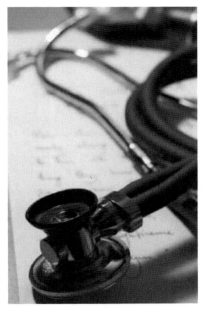

Image courtesy of a.drian via Flickr® creative commons

may be helpful in clearing bacteria in patients who are undergoing surgical procedures. The most recent study of the effect of AHCC on *K. pneumonia* was published in the *American Journal of Surgery*. In the study, researchers found that AHCC-treated mice that were infected with the bacteria were able to clear the microorganisms entirely six days after they were infected. In addition, the investigators reported that levels of important immune system cells—IL-12, IL-6 and TNF-a—peaked earlier in the AHCC group than they did in the control group. These findings led them to conclude that AHCC appears to cause an early stimulation of the immune system, which leads to an effective clearance of the disease-causing bacteria and thus results in a more rapid recovery.

AHCC Fights Fungal Infections

Candida species of fungi represent the most common fungal pathogens that can affect humans. These fungi are highly opportunistic and are responsible for a number of infections that can range from mild to deadly. Women are often familiar with candidiasis, the fungal infection caused by *Candida albicans*, because it causes a highly irritating vaginal yeast infection. However, an overgrowth of *C. albicans* can also infect other parts of the body, most notably the mouth, digestive tract and the bloodstream. When it reaches the blood, it can cause systemic infections that may cause organ failure and death.

Among the people at greatest risk of developing a *Candida* related infection are those whose immune systems are compromised by HIV/AIDS, diabetes, recent surgery, severe trauma, renal failure or organ or bone marrow transplantation; anyone who is taking antibiotics or corticosteroids; or people undergoing chemotherapy, radiation therapy, hemodialysis, parenteral hyperalimentation, catheterization or prolonged hospitalization.

Researchers at Teikyo University School of Medicine evaluated the use of AHCC in immune-compromised mice that were infected with *Candida*. One group of mice was administered 1,000 mg/kg of AHCC orally or 500 mg/kg of AHCC by injection for four days prior to their infection with *Candida*, while another group of mice did not receive AHCC. Within one week of becoming infected with *Candida*, all the control mice had died, while 80 percent of the mice injected with AHCC survived for 28 days. Oral AHCC also significantly extended survival time. When the investigators examined the mice's kidneys three days post-infection, they found that the animals treated with AHCC had one percent of the amount of yeast as the control mice.

Wrap-Up

We have shown that AHCC has proven itself to be a powerful force against many different infections. Because the results of one study found that combining AHCC with a flu vaccine improved the outcome, studies are now underway to determine the role AHCC may play as a preventive during flu season, which has the potential to be a big factor in helping people of all ages from the complications of flu. Given these findings and AHCC's great safety record (see page 63), it makes sense to consider AHCC supplementation to enhance your immune system.

Chapter 4
AHCC and Cancer

The most aggressive and far-reaching studies involving the use of AHCC have been in the area of cancer. Since the 1990s, AHCC has been used as complementary therapy in cancer patients who are undergoing conventional therapy as an immune system booster and in the process, a way to help improve their quality of life. Because AHCC was developed and registered in Japan, the vast majority of the studies have been conducted there as well. By the end of the 1990s, AHCC was being used in about 700 medical institutions, most of which were in Japan and AHCC was already accepted and used there as a food supplement for cancer because individual cases and study results suggested it was highly beneficial. In fact, AHCC became known as the "health food for cancer."

The good news is that the anticancer benefits of AHCC are being noticed and explored outside Japan, with studies in the United States at institutions such as Yale University in Connecticut, Drexel University in Philadelphia, Pennsylvania and Colorado State University, among others. Although much research remains to be done regarding the potential of AHCC in the prevention and treatment of cancer, there is a promising body of literature already available and we will review some of the work in this section. But first, let's look at the different types of cancer treatment and how AHCC differs from and fits into this scenario. Some of these studies discussed in this section have been published in journals; others have been presented at any of the International Symposium of the AHCC Research Association gatherings and/or are case reports.

Traditional Cancer Treatments

The three main conventional treatments approaches for cancer are chemotherapy, radiation therapy and surgery. All of these treatments can have a positive effect on reducing cancer, yet they also have a dramatic, detrimental impact on the immune system and the body. A fourth, up-and-coming therapy is immunotherapy, which is the category into which AHCC falls.

Chemotherapy involves the use of drugs that are toxic to both cancer cells and to normal, healthy cells. This type of cell toxicity, called cytotoxicity, affects the cells when they are dividing, which cancer cells do excessively. However, because chemotherapy also impacts healthy cells, individuals who undergo chemotherapy also experience side effects related to the damage to these cells. The cells most affected are hair root, blood and gastrointestinal tract, because all of the cells also divide rapidly. This is why chemotherapy patients typically lose their hair, experience nausea and vomiting and suffer with fatigue and increased susceptibility to infection due to damage to blood cell production. AHCC has a role to play here, as it can help alleviate symptoms associated with chemotherapy. (Read about the effect of AHCC on patients undergoing chemotherapy on page 48.)

Radiation therapy (or radiotherapy) involves the use of high-energy radiation in the form of x-rays, gamma rays and charged particles to shrink tumors and kill cancer cells. Radiation may be delivered via a machine outside the body (called external beam radiation) or from radioactive material implanted in the body (brachytherapy). Another type of radiation therapy, systemic radiation therapy, uses radioactive substances that are injected or taken by mouth and travel throughout the bloodstream to kill cancer cells. Radiation therapy kills cancer cells by destroying their DNA either directly or by creating free radicals within the cells that in turn damage the DNA. Unfortunately, radiation therapy also damages healthy cells and in the process is responsible for a variety of side effects that depend on the area of the body treated, the dose given per day, the total dose and other factors. Some of the side effects can include hair loss, urinary problems, skin irritation, fatigue, nausea and vomiting. Although some symptoms disappear when treatment stops, others can continue or late side effects may develop after treatment has ended, such as damage to the bowels that result in bleeding and diarrhea, memory loss, infertility and fibrosis.

In most cases, surgery for cancer involves removal of the tumor and some of the tissue that surrounds it. Lymph nodes are also extracted in some cases. Surgery is a major traumatic event and so has a negative impact on the immune system. Side effects associated with surgery depend mostly on the size and location of the tumor and the type of surgery performed.

Cancer Stages and Categories

Cancer Stages
Staging refers to the severity of cancer based on the extent of the original (primary) tumor and whether it has spread (metastasized) in the body. Clinicians depend on cancer staging to help them develop the most appropriate treatment for a patient, to help estimate a patient's prognosis and to determine whether patients are eligible for specific clinical trials. Because cancer staging utilizes standard terminology, it also allows healthcare providers and researchers to be "on the same page" in most cases 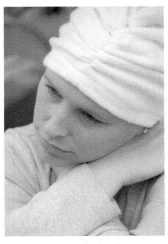 when they exchange information and compare research findings.

That said, there are differences within the staging system for the different types of cancer. For example, the criteria to assign the label "stage II" to a case of bladder cancer differs somewhat from a designation of stage II for a case of colon cancer. In addition, the prognosis for a given cancer stage depends on what kind of cancer is involved, so a stage II lung cancer has a different prognosis from a stage II cervical cancer. To help assign a cancer stage to a specific case of cancer, several elements are considered, including the site of the primary tumor, tumor size, number of tumors, involvement of the lymph nodes (spread of the cancer into lymph nodes), cell type, tumor grade and the presence or absence of metastasis.

Here is a basic outline of the stages of cancer.

Stage 0: Carcinoma *in situ*—the cancer cells are present only in the layer in which they developed

Stages I–III: The higher the number, the more extensive the disease—larger tumor sizes and/or spread of the cancer beyond the organ in which it first developed to nearby lymph nodes and/or organs near the primary tumor

Stage IV: The cancer has metastasized (spread to other organs and/or parts of the body)

As you might expect, identifying cancer stages is more complex than this and overall staging is further divided with classification such as IIA and IIB. Depending on the type of cancer, the difference in prognosis between a stage IIA and stage IIB may be very significant. Therefore, patients need to get a thorough explanation from their healthcare providers about the stage of cancer that pertains to them. Another factor that goes along with staging is tumor grade. Tumor grade is a system used to classify cancer cells in terms of how abnormal they appear under a microscope and how quickly the tumor is expected to grow and spread. The factors used to determine tumor grade are different for each type of cancer.

Cancer Categories

Cancer is also classified by category, a system that allows clinicians and researchers to use a uniform system when describing cancer and exchanging information. Those categories are:

In situ: Abnormal cells are found only in the layer of cells in which they developed

Localized: Cancer cells are present only in the organ in which they first appeared, with no evidence of spread

Regional: Cancer has spread beyond the primary site to nearby lymph nodes or organs and tissues

Distant: Cancer has spread from the primary site to distant organs or distant lymph nodes

Unknown: There is not enough information to identify the stage of cancer

Immunotherapy, BRMs and AHCC

Conventional medicine has recently added another cancer treatment modality to the mix: immunotherapy. Immunotherapy is a nontoxic method of cancer treatment that utilizes certain parts of the immune system to fight cancer or to reduce the side effects that are associated with treatment. These goals can be accomplished by stimulating the body's immune system to work harder or smarter or by taking synthetic immune system proteins or other components, known collectively as biological response modifiers (BRMs). Although immunotherapy is sometimes used alone to treat cancer, in most cases it is combined with chemotherapy or radiation therapy to enhance its effects.

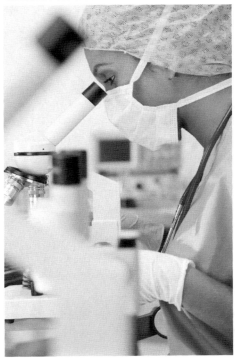

In conventional medicine, some antibodies, cytokines, vaccines and other immune system substances are synthesized in the lab to be used in cancer treatment. These BRMs change how the body's immune defenses interact with cancer cells in an attempt to enhance or restore the body's ability to fight the disease.

Does this sound familiar? If so, then you probably already know that AHCC is a biological response modifier. In fact, in Japan AHCC is widely considered to be the strongest known immune system strengthening BRM and it is often used alongside conventional cancer treatments.

When clinicians are able to halt the development of cancer using immunotherapy, a "truce" has been established between the cancer and the immune system. The cancer is dormant, and as long as the patient can maintain this state of truce, it is possible to postpone future treatment.

Following are two examples of studies that explored the impact AHCC can have on the immune systems of cancer patients.

Example One: The study was conducted at the Seoul Internal Medicine Clinic, Cancer Diagnostic Center by Dr. Jang Seok Won and included 12 cancer patients: four with stomach cancer, three with colorectal cancer, two with lung cancer and one each with breast cancer, ovarian cancer or melanoma. Won evaluated the effect of AHCC on a variety of components, including lymphocytes and NK cells, as well as various blood elements. All the patients received three to six grams of AHCC daily for three months in addition to their conventional treatment of radiotherapy or chemotherapy and they were then followed up at three, six and nine months.

Overall, Won noted the following:

- There was no significant change in white blood cell count, hemoglobin and other blood factors that would indicate a worsening of immune function, even though the patients were undergoing radiation or chemotherapy. This finding suggests AHCC can be helpful in preventing depression of bone marrow from cancer treatment.
- There was a slight increase or no change in peripheral blood lymphocytes. This was a positive sign, as lymphocyte levels tend to decrease as cancer progresses.
- The percentage of NK cells, which are important for eliminating tumor cells, increased by 21 percent after three months and was still at 20 percent six months after treatment.

Overall, AHCC appeared to be a safe and effective BRM for these cancer patients and may be helpful in preventing bone marrow depression associated with chemotherapy.

Example Two: The effects of AHCC were examined in 11 patients who had advanced cancer: three patients each with prostate, breast or ovarian cancer and two who had multiple myeloma. All the patients were treated with conventional therapies. In addition, all were administered three grams daily of AHCC. After two weeks, the researchers observed a 2.5-fold increase in the level of NK cell activity in nine of the 11 patients and the increased activity was maintained at a high level over time. They also observed a decline in PSA (prostate specific antigen) in the three prostate cancer patients. (PSA is an indicator of malignancy in prostate cancer.) Two of the three breast cancer patients showed a significant decline in the level of CA125 (cancer antigen 125), which is an antigen and a marker for this type of cancer. The rapid decrease in CA125 occurred after taking AHCC for one month and continued to decline until it reached normal values three to four months after treatment with AHCC.

The study's authors, who published their findings in the *International Journal of Immunotherapy*, also examined the impact of AHCC on tumor cell growth in two different tumor cell lines: K562 (a leukemia cell line) and Raji (a Burkitt's cell lymphoma). They found that AHCC suppressed the growth of both cell lines, with a higher concentration of AHCC (one mg/mL) providing the most effect when compared with a lower one. Overall, a one mg/mL concentration of AHCC resulted in a 21 percent reduction in the leukemia-like cell line and a 43 percent decline in the lymphoma cell line. Although the study populations in the above two studies were small, their findings suggest AHCC offers some potent anticancer activity and thus has a place in the treatment of patients who have cancer.

AHCC and Immune Surveillance

A healthy immune system performs a function called immune surveillance, in which it uncovers the presence of cancer cells and tumors throughout the body. This surveillance function is critical because cancer cells have an ability to hide, thus avoiding detection by the immune system. Restoring immune surveillance means that tumor cells can be "unmasked," which then allows the immune system to once again detect and destroy them.

White blood cells and the interferon they release are necessary for the immune system to "sniff out" and unmask cancer cells and tumors and so researchers set out to determine how AHCC may be helpful in this effort. Researchers at Yale University and Amino Up Chemical Co., Ltd. explored the effect of AHCC on immune surveillance by administering the supplement to test animals. AHCC significantly delayed the formation of melanoma and reduced tumor size. Specifically, AHCC significantly increased levels of tumor-antigen-specific immune cells and their ability to produce gamma interferon and also increased the numbers of NK cells. The authors of the study concluded that their results demonstrated that AHCC can enhance tumor immune surveillance through regulating both humoral and cell-mediated responses.

AHCC's Other Anticancer Activities

While traditional cancer treatments destroy both cancerous and healthy cells, AHCC focuses solely on the latter. That is, rather than kill cancer cells directly, AHCC strengthens and stimulates the healthy immune cells—lymphocytes, natural killer cells, macrophages and other immune compounds—whose job is to attack and/or destroy cancer cells. AHCC also improves the body's inherent immunity. AHCC can be a powerful healing force for people who have cancer.

Scores of research studies and individual case reports have illustrated the benefits associated with AHCC in patients who have cancer. Because AHCC strengthens the function of the immune system, it can be appropriate for addressing cancer that affects any part of the body. A review of the available research shows that more than 100,000 cancer patients with different types of cancer have been treated with AHCC. Results indicate that the supplement has been effective in people who have breast, colon, kidney, liver, lung, ovarian, pancreatic, stomach, testicular and tongue cancers. It appears AHCC may have an impact on cancer cells wherever they are in the body.

Overall, 60 percent of cancer patients who use AHCC along with cancer treatment have reportedly derived some benefit from the supplement. Some individuals have had a reduction in tumor mass while in others the tumor stopped growing, the cancer stopped spreading to other parts of the body, survival time increased and, in most cases, they experienced an improvement in their quality of life. For some patients, AHCC has reportedly been effective enough to induce remission from their disease.

It is important to emphasize that AHCC is used in addition to conventional cancer treatment; that is, AHCC does not replace chemotherapy, radiation therapy and/or surgery or even other immunotherapies. Doctors in Japan typically use AHCC along with mainstream cancer treatments and it is gradually gaining acceptance in other countries throughout Asia and in the United States.

AHCC and Survival from Cancer

Some studies have examined the effect of AHCC on cancer survival, including patients who are in advanced stages of the disease. For example, a total of 195 patients who were in the last stages of various cancers (e.g., gastric, colon, liver, pancreatic, lung, breast and ovarian) were given six grams of AHCC daily for six months. The patients also took other immune stimulants. The investigators monitored levels of various immune system components during the study period, including NK cells and Th1 cytokine production (e.g., interferon-gamma, IL-12). The scientists observed a significant increase in NK cell activity and in the production of interferon-gamma and IL-12, all of which support optimal immune system functioning.

Dr. Katsuaki Uno, managing director of Comfort Hospital and the head of the previously mentioned study, reported that 114 people experienced a partial or complete recovery after starting AHCC treatment. Forty percent (81 patients) experienced no change or had progression of their disease.

Although researchers often cite the immune-stimulating properties of AHCC as the reason for their helping to prolong survival from cancer, AHCC's anti-inflammatory and antistress properties have also been studied for this purpose. In the studies discussed in the following sections, you will see examples of how AHCC is associated with an improvement in quality of life and survival in cancer patients, including those with final stage or advanced disease.

AHCC and Cancer Studies

In addition to the results of other cancer studies we have already covered, several other studies have focused on one specific type of cancer and reported on the impact of AHCC in the treatment of these patients. Therefore the following cancer studies are examples of the types of research that has been done in cancer patients who included AHCC as part of their regimen for liver, gastrointestinal and breast cancer.

Liver Cancer and AHCC

Many of the cancer studies and case reports done so far have involved the use of AHCC in patients who have liver cancer. According to the World Health Organization (WHO), liver cancer is the fourth leading cause of death due to cancer (following behind lung, stomach and colorectal cancers) in the world. The American Cancer Society estimated that 24,120 adults in the United States would be diagnosed with primary liver cancer and that nearly 19,000 people would die of the disease in 2010. Liver cancer is the fifth most common cause of cancer death among men in the United States and the ninth most common among women.

Given these statistics, one would expect that the five-year relative survival rate associated with liver cancer would be poor and it is: at about 10 percent when all stages of liver cancer are considered (i.e., localized, regional and metastatic). One reason for this low survival rate is that most patients who have liver cancer also have other liver problems such as cirrhosis (scarring of the liver), which can be fatal. In patients who have small, resectable tumors (tumors that can be removed by surgery) and who do not have other liver problems, however, five-year survival can be more than 50 percent.

Generally, however, survival is poor and this is why any improvement in survival associated with the use of AHCC in liver cancer patients is especially noteworthy. Even though liver resection (surgical removal) is the most effective treatment for liver cancer, many patients are diagnosed in the late stages of the disease, when surgery would not be effective. At that point, the most commonly used treatment option is chemotherapy. However, some clinicians are also turning to BRMs and that is where AHCC can enter the picture. Two examples of AHCC's impact on liver cancer patients and survival are illustrated here.

Example One: The *Journal of Hepatology* published the results of a prospective study that covered a time span of nearly a decade, from February 1, 1992 to December 31, 2001. A total of 269 patients who had hepatocellular carcinoma were evaluated in the study. Hepatocellular carcinoma is the most common type of liver cancer and it is usually caused by cirrhosis, which can be the result of alcohol abuse, certain autoimmune diseases of the liver, hepatitis B or C, excess iron in the body (hemochromatosis) or diseases that cause long-term inflammation of the liver.

All of the patients underwent resection of the liver tumor, which is a surgical procedure to remove the affected portion of the liver. AHCC supplementation was assigned to 113 patients after surgery. The investigators noted a significantly higher overall survival rate (14 percent) among patients who took AHCC when compared with the control patients. In addition, the recurrence of cancer was significantly lower (49 percent) among the AHCC patients compared with controls (67 percent).

The mechanisms responsible for the benefits observed in the patients who took AHCC were not explored in this study. Therefore, while the authors note that AHCC intake improved liver function, reduced recurrence of liver cancer after resection and prolonged five-year survival, further research is necessary to both confirm their findings and identify the reasons behind them.

Example Two: A subsequent study was conducted in Thailand and included 44 patients with advanced liver cancer and unresectable (inoperable) tumors. All of the patients were randomly assigned to receive either AHCC (six grams daily) or a placebo until the end of their lives.

The investigators examined the patients' clinical parameters monthly or as specified to determine quality of life and various blood, biochemical and immunological parameters, such as gamma interferon and interleukin-12 levels. Magnetic resonance imaging (MRI) was performed on patients who survived longer than one year.

By week six of the study period, five (50 percent) of the patients in the placebo group had died, while all the patients in the AHCC group were alive. The follow-up period ranged from six weeks to 24 months in the AHCC group and from two weeks to 3.5 months in the control group. Overall, the median survival time was 3.5 months in the AHCC-treated patients and 1.5 months in the control patients. The investigators also noted that the percentage of lymphocytes did not decline as rapidly after AHCC treatment when compared with controls. This suggested that AHCC provided some immune system benefits for these patients in their final months. Plasma levels of IL-12 showed a slight increase in the AHCC treated patients, but it was not significant. The authors noted that their findings suggest AHCC helps to prolong the lives of patients who have advanced liver cancer. As in the previous study, the authors did not explore the mechanisms responsible for these benefits.

Gastrointestinal Cancers

Cancers of the gastrointestinal system include esophageal cancer, stomach cancer (also known as gastric cancer), colorectal cancer and anal cancer. According to the National Cancer Institute, approximately 142,570 people were diagnosed with colorectal cancer in 2010 in the United States. National Cancer Center estimates for other gastrointestinal cancers include 21,000 people diagnosed with stomach cancer, 5,260 with anal cancer and 16,640 with esophageal cancer.

Dr. Yusai Kawaguchi of the Kansai Medical University Department of Surgery in Osaka, Japan, treated two groups of cancer patients with AHCC. One group included 132 individuals with stomach cancer who took AHCC following their surgeries. Patients who had stages I–II cancer were given three grams daily of AHCC while those who had stage IV cancer took six grams per day. Patients who had stages II–IV also were taking low-dose chemotherapy.

A second group consisted of 113 patients with colon cancer. Individuals with stage I–II cancer were given three grams of AHCC daily while those with stages II–IV took six grams daily.

When the investigators compared the five-year cumulative survival rates from their two study groups with those of other institutions where AHCC was not administered, they found that in patients with stomach cancer, survival rates were superior in patients with stage I to stage IIA cancers. (Stage II stomach cancer can be classified as IIA and IIB and stage IIA has a better prognosis than does stage IIB cancer.) Among colon cancer patients with stage II and stage IIA cancer in the study, five-year cumulative survival rates were superior to those at other institutions where AHCC was not given.

Kawaguchi and his team noted that overall, use of AHCC in patients with stomach cancer and colon cancer resulted in an improvement in cumulative survival rates in some stages of cancer. These findings suggest AHCC can be beneficial as a complementary treatment for patients who have these types of cancer.

Other Cancers

In addition to all the studies we have mentioned already, there are many other individual case reports from different doctors and their experiences with patients who had pancreatic, brain, ovarian, lung, stomach, breast and other cancers and whom they treated with AHCC along with conventional treatment. Virtually without exception, the patients treated by these doctors seemed to benefit in some way from their treatment with AHCC, with an improvement in quality of life and/or pain relief being the most common advantages of taking AHCC. In some cases, patients reportedly defied their cancer and lived on for years after doctors had given up hope and beyond when conventional medicine said they would pass on.

It is important to remember, however, that AHCC is not a cure for cancer and that its place is alongside conventional treatment for cancer, as a potent immunotherapy that may provide patients with a stronger immune system and a better quality of life.

Wrap-Up

AHCC is frequently administered to patients who have cancer to strengthen, enhance and boost the immune system response, which often has the effect of improving quality of life and improving survival rates. There have been reports of patients with advanced cancer whose disease appeared to vanish after they began treatment with AHCC as a complement to conventional therapy. Any definitive relationship between use of AHCC and the disappearance of cancer in any given patient has not been determined.

Chapter 5
AHCC and Chemotherapy

More than half of the people who are diagnosed with cancer undergo chemotherapy at some point. This means tens of millions of children and adults are treated each year with drugs designed to kill cancer cells, but these drugs also destroy healthy cells and as a result cause some significant side effects, as noted in the previous section. Some cancer cells grow slowly while others grow rapidly, therefore clinicians need to select different chemotherapy drugs designed to target the specific growth patterns of a person's cancer cells. Whether the drugs taken are designed to attack cancer cells that grow slowly or rapidly, medication-related complications are often a result.

Of the common side effects associated with chemotherapy—nausea and vomiting, hair loss, fatigue, impaired liver function, loss of appetite and low levels of white blood cells, 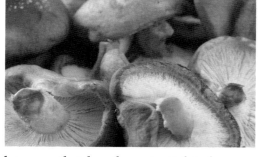 red blood cells and platelets, one that has the potential to be very serious is *neutropenia,* or low white blood cell levels. White blood cells fight infections and if patients' levels drop too low, they may need to stop chemotherapy for a while. This action not only places patients at an increased risk for serious infections that could be life-threatening, but it also interrupts their cancer treatment.

Impaired liver function also can be dangerous and infrequently can result in liver failure. Low platelet levels (thrombocytopenia) could result in clotting problems (e.g., easy or excessive bruising, excessive bleeding when cut, bloody nose or gums, blood in the urine), while low red blood cells levels often cause anemia, characterized by fatigue, dizziness and shortness of breath.

Given the great number of cancer patients who undergo chemotherapy each year and the disruptive and sometimes debilitating side effects it can cause, it is important that these individuals have effective options available to them to help alleviate and possibly eliminate these adverse effects and enhance their quality of life. AHCC supplementation has demonstrated an ability to help chemotherapy patients improve their lives in some of the ways we discuss here.

Hair Loss

Losing one's hair because of chemotherapy is not a life-threatening side effect, but it can be very life-altering and emotionally devastating. Both men and women report that hair loss is one of the side effects they most fear after they are diagnosed with cancer. Not everyone who undergoes chemotherapy loses their hair, because it depends on the type and dose of drug used. However, hair root cells grow rapidly and if you have a rapidly growing cancer, chances are you can expect to lose hair and not just from your scalp. Chemotherapy can cause eyebrow, armpit, pubic, eyelash and other body hair to fall out.

The good news is that in most cases, hair loss from chemotherapy is temporary: hair tends to regrow three to 10 months after treatment ends. The other good news is that AHCC may help reduce hair loss.

For example, scientists evaluated the effect of AHCC on hair loss caused by a single dose of the chemotherapy drug cytosine arabinoside (Ara-C). Rats used in the study were administered either 500 mg/kg per day of AHCC for seven consecutive days plus a single dose of Ara-C or a single dose of Ara-C. Results of the study, which were published in *Cancer Epidemiology* in 2009, showed that five of seven rats treated with Ara-C alone had severe hair loss and two had moderate hair loss. Four of the nine rats that received both Ara-C and AHCC, however, experienced mild hair loss, while four had moderate hair loss and one had severe hair loss.

Nausea and Vomiting

According to the American Cancer Society, nausea and vomiting are among the most feared side effects of chemotherapy. Even though these symptoms are not considered life-threatening, they can significantly disrupt the lives of those who experience them, making it very difficult or impossible for them to work, care for their children and perform normal, everyday functions.

Although the prevalence and severity of nausea and vomiting associated with chemotherapy have been somewhat alleviated by the introduction of new drugs to treat these symptoms, such drugs are not for everyone. Some patients do not want to take additional drugs along with their chemotherapy. In addition, anti-nausea drugs are not always effective and may also have side effects of their own, which can add to the discomfort cancer patients experience. Nausea and vomiting can be so severe for some cancer patients that they choose to stop their chemotherapy.

Clinical studies and case reports show that AHCC can improve patients' quality of life regarding nausea and vomiting. In one small study, for example, Dr. G.H. Ahn of Ok-Cherm Hospital in South Korea prescribed AHCC for eight months to 12 patients who had stage II–IV cancer. Over the treatment period Dr. Ahn noted any changes in nausea, vomiting and pain experienced by the patients and found an improvement in all three symptoms, which results in a better quality of life for these patients.

Impaired Liver and Spleen Function

In the same study that explored the effect of AHCC on hair loss in rats exposed to a chemotherapy drug, researchers also evaluated the impact of AHCC on modulating liver damage. To accomplish this, they administered a single dose of 6-mercaptopurine (6-MP) plus methotrexate (MTX), two antimetabolite, cancer-fighting drugs, to two groups of rats: one group received the drugs only and a second group received AHCC for 28 days plus a single dose of 6-MP plus MTX.

The researchers then measured the levels of two liver enzymes that are used to determine the degree of liver function: SGOT (serum glutamic oxaloacetic transaminase, also called aspartate transaminase) and SGPT (serum glutamic pyruvate transaminase, also called alanine transaminase). The higher the levels of these enzymes, the greater the damage and destruction to liver tissue. The scientists found that rats given AHCC had normal levels of SGOT and SGPT while the untreated rats had large increases in these enzyme levels.

In addition, the rats treated with AHCC along with 6-MP and MTX demonstrated significantly increased body weight and levels of leukocytes and red blood cells. All these factors together indicated that AHCC significantly reduced the side effects associated with the chemotherapy drugs.

The spleen is an organ that people don't hear much about, but it plays an important role in immune function. This fist-sized organ is part of the lymphatic system, contains white blood cells that fight infections and destroys damaged and old cells. Although it is true that people can live without a spleen, the body loses some of its ability to fight infections if the spleen is removed because of disease or damage.

A team of scientists investigated the impact of AHCC on the spleen after it was subjected to chemotherapy. The researchers used the chemotherapy drug cyclophosphamide, which typically causes the spleen to shrink in size by 50 percent. In mouse models, the researchers noted that the spleens in mice given cyclophosphamide plus AHCC did not shrink as much as they did in mice not treated with AHCC. The AHCC-treated mice also had a lower rate of infection than mice not treated with AHCC.

Myelosuppression

Chemotherapy can both destroy white blood cells as well as damage bone marrow function, a condition also known as myelosuppression. Bone marrow is the spongy tissue located inside some large bones that houses stem cells. These stem cells transform themselves into white and red blood cells and platelets. When chemotherapy damages bone marrow, the production and levels of these critical immune system substances decline. The result is that patients become highly susceptible to infections and they may also develop anemia, which exacerbates their lowered resistance. Overall, myelosuppression is a very serious and life-threatening state.

Several studies have shown that AHCC can have a positive effect on myelosuppression and improve the white blood cell levels in response to chemotherapy. In South Korea, Dr. G.H. Ahn of

Ok-Cherm Hospital administered six grams daily of AHCC to 12 patients who had stage II–IV cancer (two patients each had breast, ovarian, stomach, lung, uterine and lung cancers) and who were undergoing chemotherapy. Over a period of seven months, levels of white blood cells rose from below 6,000 to nearly 8,000.

In animal studies, scientists have observed a reduction in damage to bone marrow when AHCC was administered. In one such study, published in *Cancer Epidemiology*, two chemotherapy drugs (cyclophosphamide and 5-fluorouracil) were given to four groups of mice: one group each received one of the drugs, one group received AHCC plus cyclophosphamide and one group received AHCC plus 5-fluorouracil. The red blood cell count remained close to normal in the two groups of mice that were treated with AHCC, but it declined in the two groups that received the chemotherapy drugs only. A study in rats given chemotherapy also demonstrated that oral intake of AHCC protected the animals against a loss of red blood cell production.

Similar results were observed in another mouse study reported in *AHCC: Research and Commentary* that used four groups of mice. Two groups were injected with chemotherapy drugs (5-fluorouracil and cyclophosphamide, methotrexate and 6-mercaptopurine) alone and the other two received the drugs plus AHCC. Mice that received AHCC had a normal weight and normal levels of red blood cells, while the mice not treated with AHCC expressed a decline in both of these factors. Although the AHCC-treated mice showed some decline in white blood cell counts, it was not as significant as the decline observed in the drug-only groups.

In a study published in the *Journal of Experimental Therapeutics & Oncology*, scientists evaluated the impact of AHCC in groups of mice that were treated with a variety of chemotherapy regimens, including paclitaxel alone or some combination of paclitaxel, 5-fluorouracil, cisplatin, irinotecan, doxorubicin and/or cyclophosphamide. They found that the myelosuppressive effects of chemotherapy were generally alleviated in mice that also received AHCC and that both liver and kidney toxicity related to chemotherapy were significantly improved by AHCC.

The ability of AHCC to mitigate myelosuppression and to enhance immune cell activity and function are critically important benefits for individuals who experience a decline in white blood cell levels as a result of chemotherapy, as well as a potential way to reduce the risks associated with this life-threatening complication.

Loss of Appetite

Along with nausea and vomiting, chemotherapy can cause cancer patients to experience changes in taste. These factors often add up to a loss of appetite and poor nutritional intake. Because cancer patients already have a compromised immune system, a poor or inadequate diet can result in weight loss, a breakdown in muscle, increased susceptibility to infection and an overall poorer quality of life.

AHCC has been used by thousands of cancer patients and many report an improvement in loss of appetite when taking the supplement while undergoing chemotherapy. When their appetite is restored, patients are better able to maintain or regain lost weight, improve their nutritional intake and support their immune system.

Is AHCC Safe to Use with Chemotherapy?

The answer, with one caveat, is yes. In fact, AHCC is reported to enhance and strengthen the therapeutic effects of the anticancer agent cisplatin, paclitaxel, doxorubicin and perhaps others as well. The caveat relates to the results of a study conducted by Dr. Judith A. Smith and published in the *Journal of the Society for Integrative Oncology*. Researchers found that AHCC may be involved in a drug-drug interaction when used with chemotherapy agents that are metabolized via a specific pathway called CYP450 2D6. This includes drugs such as tamoxifen. Specifically, use of AHCC with these drugs may reduce the effectiveness of these drugs. The authors concluded that "the overall data suggest that AHCC would be safe to administer with most other chemotherapy agents that are not metabolized via the CYP450 2D6 pathway."

Wrap-Up

The take-home message here is that AHCC has demonstrated the ability to improve the quality of life of patients who are plagued with side effects associated with chemotherapy. This is no small achievement, as people with cancer often feel like they are losing control of their health and their lives. Making the functional food AHCC a part of their treatment plan can provide them with a safe, natural way to improve the quality of their lives while they battle cancer.

Chapter 6
Other Chronic Diseases

The ability of AHCC to have a positive impact on immune cells and immune response throughout the body opens the door for its use in treating many health challenges. Research into the numerous possibilities is ongoing and thus far scientists have documented promising results, which we share with you in this section.

Diabetes

Diabetes is a formidable opponent and the statistics on the prevalence, future projections and complications regarding type 2 diabetes are alarming. Data from the American Diabetes Association in 2011 reported that 25.8 million children and adults in the United States—nearly eight percent of the population—have diabetes. An additional 79 million have pre-diabetes, which means they are very likely to develop the full-blown disease within a few years. Each year, 1.9 million new cases of diabetes are diagnosed in people aged 20 years and older. In 2010, the CDC forecasted that as many as one in three people (33 percent) in the United States could have diabetes by 2050, more than triple the current number.

The complications associated with diabetes are often debilitating and deadly. Adults with diabetes have heart disease death rates that are two to four times higher than adults without diabetes and the same higher risk applies to stroke as well. Diabetes is the leading cause of new cases of blindness among adults and it is also the main cause of kidney failure. About 75 percent of adults with diabetes have blood pressure greater than or equal to 130/80 mmHg or take prescription medication for hypertension and between 60 and 70 percent of people with diabetes have nervous system damage (neuropathy).

Research indicates that both inflammation and oxidative stress (a state in which the body has an excess amount of free radicals and/or an insufficient level of antioxidants to fight them) are involved in type 2 diabetes. In addition, inflammation appears to hinder the body's ability to properly utilize insulin as well as contribute to the breakdown in the cells that produce insulin in the pancreas. AHCC has anti-inflammatory properties, so scientists have explored its use in animal models of diabetes.

In a study conducted at Dokkyo University School of Medicine in Saitama, Japan, Dr. Koji Wakame used rats with diabetes induced with the drug streptozotocin. One group of rats were pretreated with AHCC for one week before they were given streptozotocin while a second group of rats did not receive AHCC. The untreated rats lost weight and their fur, increased their intake of water, had markers associated with a stressed liver and demonstrated a decline in insulin levels accompanied by a rise in blood sugar levels—all signs of diabetes.

The AHCC-treated rats did not lose their fur, gained a small amount of weight, had no increase in water intake, had normal liver markers and maintained normal insulin and blood sugar levels. Upon microscopic examination, Wakame observed a decline in the number of insulin-producing cells in the pancreas in the untreated rats and only a slight decline in the AHCC-treated rats. Wakame concluded that AHCC may have a significant effect in preventing the onset of diabetes by protecting the insulin-producing cells.

In another study, presented at the 12th International Symposium of the AHCC Research Association in 2004, researchers at Osaka University in Osaka, Japan, also used rats with diabetes induced by streptozotocin. They reported that AHCC suppressed the onset of diabetes and delayed the development of complications.

Dr. M. Iwamoto of Nobuyama Medical Corporation conducted a study that involved 13 diabetic patients. All the individuals took AHCC for more than six months and experienced significant declines in both average blood glucose levels and glycohemoglobin. This latter factor is measured in a test called the glycohemoglobin A1c. The glycohemoglobin A1c level is important because, unlike a blood glucose level which is a "snapshot" of how well a person is controlling his or her diabetes, it provides clinicians with a reliable indication of how well the diabetes has been controlled over the last two to three months.

Two patients from Dr. Iwamoto's study can serve as examples of what is possible with AHCC in diabetes. He reported that when a patient who has a blood sugar level of 250 mg/dL (normal is 70 to 110 mg/dL) take AHCC, blood sugar levels often return to normal after six months' treatment with AHCC. In these same patients, who often have glycohemoglobin A1c level of 9.1 percent (normal is four to six percent), glycohemoglobin A1c levels can decline to 6.8 percent. In a patient whose glycohemoglobin A1c declined to six percent after taking AHCC for one month, the blood sugar level decreased to a normal value after two months of AHCC. In the latter patient, glycohemoglobin A1c levels remained normal and a problem with paralysis of the left leg associated with diabetic neuropathy improved.

Liver Diseases

Previously, we noted that AHCC may help prevent liver damage in cancer patients who are receiving chemotherapy. Other reports suggest AHCC may be helpful in treating serious liver diseases, such as acute liver failure and hepatitis. Acute liver failure is an uncommon but serious condition that has a high mortality rate. "Hepatitis" means inflammation of the liver and it also refers to a group of viruses that affect the organ. The most common types are hepatitis A, B and C. According to the CDC, in 2008, an estimated 4.4 million Americans were living with chronic hepatitis, although most of them are not aware they are infected. Approximately 80,000 new infections occur each year in the United States.

Some studies of AHCC in liver disease have demonstrated promising results. For example, a mouse study was conducted to identify the effect of AHCC on liver damage. A group of mice were given AHCC in advance of being treated with carbon tetrachloride, which is known to cause liver damage and in animal studies has been shown to increase the risk of liver cancer. The scientists discovered that AHCC prevented a decline in the enzyme glutathione S-transferase (GST), which is involved in detoxification. Therefore, AHCC reduced the amount of liver damage associated with carbon tetrachloride. In addition, when the scientists studied liver cells from the mice under a microscope, they found that cell destruction had been prevented. Overall, the researchers concluded that AHCC prevented damage to the liver associated with the oxidation caused by a toxin such as carbon tetrachloride.

Acute liver failure, which includes both fulminant liver failure (which causes coma within two weeks of onset of symptoms) and subfulminant liver failure (or late-onset liver failure, which causes coma within two weeks to three months after onset of symptoms) is an uncommon condition in which the liver undergoes rapid deterioration in a previously health individual. The condition usually affects young people and has a high mortality rate ranging from 60 to 80 percent. Scientists explored the effect of AHCC in an animal model of acute liver failure.

In the experiment, which was conducted by Professor Masatoshi Yamazaki of Teikyo University's Department of Pharmacy, two groups of mice were administered lipopolysaccharides (LPS) and galactosamine to induce acute liver failure: one group was pretreated with AHCC and the other group was not. Thirty percent (three out of 10) mice that did not receive AHCC died within 24 hours of receiving LPS and galactosamine while none of the AHCC-treated mice died. Thus, the researchers concluded that AHCC protected the mice against drug-induced liver failure.

Experts have also looked at possible benefits of AHCC in hepatitis patients. In some cases of hepatitis and liver cancer, patients and doctors report an improvement in the loss of platelets, a decrease or elimination of the viral load (the concentration of virus in the blood) and cessation of the deterioration of liver function.

An example of how AHCC may help patients with hepatitis can be seen in a case study of a 32-year-old man who had chronic hepatitis B. After he began taking three grams of AHCC daily, he experienced a decline in the HBe antigen value (which indicates the amount of hepatitis B virus) and his HBe antibody value (the antibody that helps eliminate the hepatitis B virus) increased. Although the patient's platelet count decreased even after he started taking AHCC, it did not continue to decline. Eventually, elimination of the hepatitis B virus was confirmed.

People with hepatitis C also reportedly respond to AHCC. Hepatitis C is a chronic viral infection that is characterized by elevated levels of liver enzymes, high viral loads, inflammation and scarring of the liver. Untreated hepatitis C can result in cirrhosis and liver cancer.

Healthcare professionals, especially in Asia, have reported on case studies in which three to six grams of AHCC daily have reduced liver enzyme levels and other chronic diseases loads in hepatitis C patients. Other reports indicate that numerous patients have achieved a decline in viral load of more than 80 percent after taking AHCC for six months and that some reach the normal viral load range after taking AHCC for seven to 12 months. Controlled studies are still needed to verify these findings.

Cardiovascular Disease

Cardiovascular diseases are the leading cause of death in the United States. According to the latest available figures from the American Heart Association, more than 81 million people in the United States have some form of cardiovascular disease (e.g., hypertension, coronary heart disease, stroke, heart failure) and approximately 34 percent of all deaths are attributed to a form of heart disease.

AHCC possesses a few qualities that may help in the prevention of cardiovascular disease. One is via its anti-inflammatory properties, as scientists have identified inflammation as playing a key role in cardiovascular disease. As we discussed in the first section, CRP levels are an indication of the amount of inflammation in the body and blood levels of CRP are a sign of increased risk of stroke, heart attack and other cardiovascular conditions. AHCC has demonstrated an ability to reduce CRP levels.

Another way AHCC may benefit the cardiovascular system is through its ability to increase the production of nitric oxide. Nitric oxide is a chemical produced in the inner lining of the blood vessels (endothelium). Enzymes convert the amino acid arginine and oxygen into nitric oxide through a series of steps.

Nitric oxide is important to heart health because it relaxes the smooth muscle in blood vessels, which improves the flow of blood. It may also widen blood vessels and arteries, which in turn can reduce the amount of pressure exerted onto the vessel walls by the blood. Nitric oxide's antioxidant properties can reduce the buildup of plaque in the arteries by lowering cholesterol and calming inflammation that causes plaque to accumulate.

One challenge presented by nitric oxide is that while high levels in the blood seem to reduce the risk of cardiovascular disease, there are few dietary or lifestyle factors that can impact nitric oxide production. AHCC may be able to address that challenge.

Other Conditions

Given the many positive results AHCC has shown in the host of studies regarding enhancement of immune function, it appears that AHCC may be beneficial in the treatment of many other ailments and diseases, although clinical studies specifically for this purpose have not yet been conducted.

- **Arthritis:** Given AHCC's anti-inflammatory properties, for example, it may help individuals who suffer with arthritis. Dr. Mitsuaki Iwamoto of the Enzankai Medical Corporation in Japan reports that patients with rheumatoid arthritis who have taken AHCC continuously experience an improvement in their symptoms. This may be the result of AHCC's ability to stimulate a reduction in levels of TNF-a and a substance called calprotectin, both of which have pro-inflammatory properties. Calprotectin is found in large amounts in the synovial fluid around the joints in patients who have rheumatoid arthritis.

- **Amyotrophic lateral sclerosis:** In a mouse model of ALS (amyotrophic lateral sclerosis), a progressive disease that affects the muscles and eventually results in death, scientists tested the possible benefits of AHCC in treating this autoimmune disease. In mice with laboratory-induced ALS, the administration of AHCC significantly enhanced grip strength and survival. This finding was presented at the 12th International Symposium of the AHCC Research Association.

- **Colitis:** Colitis is a type of inflammatory bowel disease characterized by inflammation of the colon. Investigators in Spain induced the disease using hapten in two groups of rats. In one group, however, the animals were pretreated with AHCC. The rats pretreated with AHCC showed significantly lower levels of pro-inflammatory cytokines compared with the untreated rats.

- **HIV/AIDS:** According to anecdotal reports regarding patients with HIV, AHCC is reported to maintain T cell counts and even increase them in some cases. This is critically important in people who have HIV, which attacks T cells. Dr. Daniel Rubin, a naturopathic physician board certified in naturopathic oncology, reportedly has prescribed AHCC for AIDS patients and confirmed an increase in B-lymphocytes and CD8+. Reports regarding AIDS patients claim AHCC increased T cell counts after just one month of treatment, accompanied by an increase in the activity of NK cells, which typically are weakened in people who have HIV.

- **Glaucoma:** People suffering with glaucoma have noted a reduction in intraocular pressure (pressure in the fluid in the eye).

- **Hypertension:** AHCC has been associated with lowering blood pressure in people with hypertension.

- **Chronic Fatigue Syndrome:** Individuals with chronic fatigue syndrome have reported an improvement in fatigue after taking AHCC. Dr. Dan Kenner, PhD, LAc (licensed acupuncturist), recommends three grams of AHCC daily for at least six weeks for treatment of chronic fatigue syndrome.

Wrap-Up

Despite more than two decades of research, the full scope of benefits people can reap from AHCC has hardly been realized. Significant inroads into its impact on diabetes, cardiovascular disease, liver diseases and other chronic illnesses have already been made. Because AHCC can impact the body's immunity at a very basic level, the possibilities appear to be quite substantial.

Chapter 7
Using AHCC

Now that you have read about the research surrounding the use of AHCC and the various beneficial effects it can have on the immune system, you are probably wondering how to use AHCC —how much to take and who can use it—as well as any side effects, its safety record and if it can be taken with other medications. All these questions and more are covered in this section.

Taking AHCC

AHCC is manufactured by only one company, Amino Up Chemical Co., Ltd., and is available as fine granules, soft granules in capsules and as a liquid. AHCC should be taken orally only, never by injection.

If you are in good health and want to take AHCC as a preventive measure and/or to maintain your health, then one to three grams daily is suggested. This can be taken as two to six 500 mg capsules. If you are undergoing treatment for cancer (chemotherapy, radiation therapy, surgery), then three to six grams daily is recommended while cancer treatment is ongoing. This dosage can be reduced to three grams daily after treatment has ended to help prevent recurrence of cancer. In either case, it is best to take AHCC in divided doses three times a day (e.g., one to two grams three times daily).

Children can take AHCC as well, but you should reduce the dosage by up to 50 percent because of lower body weight. For elderly patients, the dose should be moderated to match their physical condition and introduced gradually as older individuals may have hypersensitive digestive systems. AHCC can be mixed with yogurt or honey to make it easier to consume.

Although AHCC has no reported side effects when taken in appropriate amounts or when taken with conventional medications or supplements, consult a healthcare provider before taking AHCC yourself or giving it to a child or other adult, especially if you or the other individuals are taking any prescription or over-the-counter (OTC) medications or supplements.

Quality and Safety

AHCC is manufactured by only one company and under a strict, proprietary production method and culturing system. The manufacturing methods prevent contamination from foreign microorganisms and facilitate a stable culturing environment for the entire process. The manufacturers use computer monitoring to help ensure culture conditions (e.g., temperature, stirring, etc.) are always properly controlled.

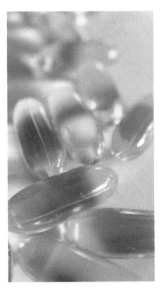

Generally, health foods derived from mushrooms are natural products, which means the components may differ depending on the producer and how the products are manufactured. When AHCC is produced, however, the chemical constituents and the quality are consistently maintained through attention to every detail of the manufacturing process and the latest technology.

Since AHCC was first developed in 1983, safety studies have been conducted according to standards equivalent to the Good Manufacturing Practices (GMPs), standards for clinical research protocols on the safety of medicines. GMPs provide standards for toxicity tests in animal testing. Along with general toxicity tests, standards for special toxicity tests (such as reproduction/generation tests, carcinogenesis tests and others) have also been developed. Despite the use of doses in excess of those estimated to be fatal in animals, AHCC has not demonstrated any toxicity.

In 1994, the AHCC Research Association was established. This association consists of professionals from medical institutions and universities who are working to prove AHCC's medical reliability. Thus far, researchers have produced volumes of reports on basic research and studies related to clinical and safety issues. Dozens of studies have been published in journals, while scores of case reports have been documented. Although much work remains to be done, the results thus far have been very promising and thousands of patients have benefited from taking AHCC.

Taking AHCC with Other Medications

Research, including evaluations done by Dr. Judith A. Smith, has shown that AHCC can be taken along with most conventional medications without initiating any drug-supplement interactions. This includes chemotherapy drugs and supportive therapies, such as antidepressants and anti-nausea medications, as well as insulin and OTC drugs.

There is one minor exception. AHCC can induce an enzyme called CYP450 2D6, which is involved in certain metabolic processes. If AHCC is taken with drugs such as Ondansetron (Zofran–often used to treat chemotherapy-induced nausea and vomiting) or Sertraline (Zoloft-a common antidepressant), which are substrates of this enzyme, it may decrease the activity of these drugs. Therefore, consult a physician before using AHCC if you are using any medications, both prescription and OTC, as well as any supplements.

Natural Ways to Enhance Your Immune System

Although AHCC is proving to be an excellent way to enhance and strengthen the immune system, it is unreasonable to expect that taking AHCC is all you need to do to protect yourself against illness and disease. Numerous lifestyle habits and other factors are also essential for achieving and maintaining an optimally functioning immune system. Those factors include the following:

- **Get regular exercise.** Studies show that participating in regular moderate exercise (such as 30 minutes of brisk walking or bicycling) four to five times a week boosts the immune system by raising the level of infection-fighting white blood cells. Inactivity can weaken the immune system indirectly by contributing to obesity, poor sleep and other problems that can increase risk of disease.

- **Maintain a healthy weight.** Being overweight or obese increases the risk of developing heart disease, cancer, diabetes and other serious conditions. An excessive number of fat cells can trigger the release of pro-inflammatory chemicals that can result in chronic inflammation that leads to tissue damage and disease. Animal studies have shown that being overweight or obese causes a reduction in the number of antibodies the body produces after receiving vaccinations.

- **Manage stress.** Short-term stress may actually help the immune system operate better. In response to stress, the body produces cortisol, the "fight or flight" hormone that helps resolve the stressful situation. Chronic stress, however, can be damaging to the immune system, as the steady release of stress hormones, including cortisol and adrenaline, suppresses the system's ability to ward off infections and disease. Epidemiological (population) research into health psychology suggests there is a high risk of cancer in people who experience high levels of emotional stress. To help manage stress, choose management techniques that work best for you, whether that is exercise, meditation, aromatherapy, psychological counseling, yoga, dancing, deep breathing, laughter or visualization, among others. Such methods have been studied to varying degrees regarding their ability to help individuals reduce and manage stress.

- **Follow a nutritious diet.** A diet that focuses on antioxidant-rich foods (such as fresh fruits and vegetables, whole grains and legumes) supports the immune system. Antioxidants neutralize the cell-damaging molecules called free radicals, which can contribute to cancer and other diseases. Other immune supporting foods include fresh garlic, turmeric and mushrooms. A nutritious diet also means minimizing or avoiding sugars and unhealthy fats, such as saturated and trans fats. For example, consuming 75 to 100 grams of a sugar solution daily, which is equal to two 12-ounce soft drinks, can suppress the body's ability to respond to immune system challenges. Table sugar, fructose, glucose and honey can all cause white blood cells to lose 50 percent of their ability to digest bacteria.

- **Stay socially connected.** Building and maintaining strong relationships and social networks is critical for both physical and emotional health. Studies show that people who feel they have a good social network have a stronger immune system than people who feel alone.

- **Get adequate sleep.** Fatigue feeds illness: when you have not been getting enough sleep, you are more likely to develop an infection. Insomnia can cause a rise in cortisol levels, which in turn can lead to inflammation. Adults should get seven to eight hours of sleep per night for good health.

- **Avoid environmental toxins.** This can be a tough one, given the many ways people are exposed to chemicals and pollutants in air, water, food, soil and everyday consumer products. A good start: avoid food additives, use natural cleaning products in your home and on the job, use natural pest control products in your garden, avoid secondhand smoke, use filtered water, buy organic foods when possible, avoid dry cleaning and use a natural soap to wash your hands often.

Chapter 8
Q&A

Q: *Is AHCC only for people who are sick, or can someone who is generally healthy take it to boost their immune system?*
A: AHCC's potent antioxidant properties may provide the immune system boost many people need in today's high-powered, overly stressed world. For individuals who are generally in good health and who want to support and maintain their immune system, one to three grams of AHCC per day is typically sufficient and recommended as an "insurance policy" against unexpected and unwelcome bacteria, viruses, environmental toxins and other assaults to the immune system.

Q: *Can AHCC be used instead of conventional cancer treatments?*
A: AHCC is not a cure for cancer and therefore anyone with cancer should take advantage of the many conventional treatment options for cancer. However, AHCC is suggested as a complementary treatment for anyone who is preparing to undergo conventional cancer treatment, as well as patients who are currently in treatment and for those who have completed treatment. AHCC can offer immune system enhancing benefits to individuals in each of these circumstances.

Q: *If AHCC is made from mushrooms, why can't I just eat mushrooms and get the same benefits?*
A: Although whole mushrooms do possess many beneficial nutrients, AHCC is the product of special processing and culturing of selected mushrooms to produce a functional food that has a unique constituent called acylated alpha-glucan. Alpha-glucan has a low molecular weight that makes it easy for the body to digest and

absorb. These unique components also have a powerful immune-stimulating action not found in ordinary mushrooms, or in other mushroom products.

Q: *Does immunity (cell-mediated immunity) improve in everyone who takes AHCC?*
A: Although the studies conducted thus far have shown that use of AHCC can result in an improvement in immunity for many patients suffering from various diseases and for healthy individuals as well, not everyone responds in the same way or to the same degree. Therefore, there is no guarantee AHCC will strengthen your immune system. The immune system is a complex network and a compromised immune system is especially so. Strengthening and supporting one's immune system defenses is a job that requires many helpers. AHCC is just one of such helpers, albeit a potent one.

Q: *Besides AHCC, are there other natural immune system boosters?*
A: Although many other nutritional and herbal supplements are used to boost the immune system, AHCC has probably undergone more intensive research than all of them. However, others to consider include astragalus, echinacea, flavonoids (plant compounds such as quercetin and catechins [found in green tea]), garlic, goldenseal, maitake (a Chinese mushroom), probiotics (beneficial bacteria), reishi (another Chinese mushroom), vitamins C, D and E and zinc. Before taking these and any other supplements, consult a knowledgeable healthcare professional.

Q: *Can AHCC be used in companion animals, such as dogs and cats?*
A: For many people, dogs and cats are considered members of the family and when these animals develop serious health conditions such as cancer, some individuals turn to veterinary specialists who can offer them a variety of treatment options to improve their pet's quality of life and to treat symptoms. Numerous reports of the use of AHCC in dogs and cats have been recorded. Assistant professor Masato Kuwahara of Nihon University's Department of Veterinary Radiation Research located in Tokyo, Japan, and a colleague evaluated the use of AHCC and shark cartilage on breast cancer tumors in dogs. This combination was used because AHCC is an immune system stimulator and shark cartilage is an angiogenesis

inhibitor (prevents the formation of new blood vessels that feed tumors, thus starving them). A total of 62 dogs that had breast cancer were given these two supplements twice daily for more than 60 days. The combination had an antitumor effect in 29 dogs and improved quality of life in 45. Progression of the tumor was stopped in 24 dogs.

In addition to this study, individual veterinarians have used either AHCC plus shark cartilage or AHCC alone in dogs with breast and other cancers. There are also reports that AHCC is effective against age-related diseases, such as cataracts.

Suggested dosage for animals are as follows:

Suggested Pet Dosage Range

Size	Maintenance Dose per day	Therapeutic Dose per day
Large Pet (75lbs)	500 mgs-1 gram	1.5 grams to 3 grams
Small Pet (32lbs)	250-500 mgs	750 mgs-1.5 grams

Q: *Where can I get more information about AHCC?*
A: The AHCC Research Association's website, www.ahccresearch.com, provides information about the functional food, including research articles, presented studies and general information about AHCC.

References

AHCC: A Most Remarkable Mushroom

Uno, K. et al. "Active hexose correlated compound (AHCC) improves immunological parameters and performance status of patients with solid tumors." *Biotherapy* 14, no. 3 (May 2000): 303–309.

Yui, S. "Suppressive effect of AHCC on acute inflammation." AHCC Research Association 7th Symposium, Sapporo, Japan, 1999 and 2000.

Introducing Your Immune System

Aviles H., T. Belay et al. "Active hexose correlated compound enhances resistance to *Klebsiella pneumonia* infection in mice in the hind limb-unloading model of spaceflight conditions." *Journal of Applied Physiology* 95, no. 2 (August 2003): 491–6.

Aviles, H., P. O'Donnell et al. "Active hexose correlated compound activates immune function to decrease bacterial load in a murine model of intramuscular infection." *American Journal of Surgery* 195, no. 4 (April 2008): 537–45.

————. "Active hexose correlated compound (AHCC) enhances resistance to infection in a mouse model of surgical wound infection." *Surgical Infections* 7, no. 6 (December 2006): 527–35.

Ishibashi H., T. Ikeda, et al. "Prophylactic efficacy of a basiodiomycetes preparation AHCC against lethal opportunistic infections in mice." *Yakugaku Zasshi: Journal of the Pharmaceutical Society of Japan* 120, no. 8 (August 2000): 715–9.

Spierlings E.L., H. Fujii, et al. "A phase I study of the safety of the nutritional supplement, active hexose correlated compound, AHCC, in healthy volunteers." *Journal of Nutritional Science and Vitaminology* 53, no. 6 (December 2007): 536–9.

Terakawa N. Y. Matsui, et al. "Immunological effect of active hexose correlated compound (AHCC) in healthy volunteers: a double-blind, placebo-controlled trial." *Nutrition and Cancer* 60, no. 5 (2008): 643–51.

Yin Z., et al. "Determining the frequency of CD4+ and CD8+ T cells producing IFN gamma and TNF-a in healthy elderly people using flow cytometry before and after AHCC intake." *Human Immunology* 71, no. 12 (December 2010): 1187–90.

Colds, Flu and Other Infections

Aviles H., T. Belay et al. "Active hexose correlated compound enhances resistance to *Klebsiella pneumonia infection* in mice in the hindlimb-unloading model of spaceflight conditions." *Journal of Applied Physiology* 95, no. 2 (August 2003): 491–6.

Aviles, H., P. O'Donnell et al. "Active hexose correlated compound activates immune function to decrease bacterial load in a murine model of intramuscular infection." *American Journal of Surgery* 195, no. 4 (April 2008): 537–45.

———. "Active hexose correlated compounds (AHCC) enhances resistance to infection in a mouse model of surgical wound infection." *Surgical Infections* 7, no. 6 (December 2006): 527–35.

Fujii H., H. Nishioka, et al. "Nutritional food active hexose correlated compound (AHCC) enhances resistance against bird flu." *Japanese Journal of Complementary and Alternative Medicine* 4, no. 2 (2007): 37–9.

Ishibashi H., T. Ikeda, et al. "Prophylactic efficacy of a basiodiomycetes preparation AHCC against lethal opportunistic infections in mice." *Yakugaku Zasshi: Journal of the Pharmaceutical Society of Japan* 120, no. 8 (August 2000): 715–9.

Ritz B.W., S. Nogusa, et al. "Supplementation with active hexose correlated compound increases the innate immune response of young mice to primary influenza infection." *Journal of Nutrition* 136, no. 11 (November 2006): 2868–73.

Wang S., T. Welte, et al. "Oral administration of active hexose correlated compound enhances host resistance to West Nile encephalitis in mice." *Journal of Nutrition* 139, no. 3 (March 2009): 598–602.

Centers for Disease Control and Prevention. "West Nile Virus: What You Need To Know." 2006. http://www.cdc.gov/ncidod/dvbid/westnile/wnv_factsheet.htm.

Todar, K. "Opportunistic Infections Caused by *Pseudomonas aeruginosa.*" University of Wisconsin-Madison. 2009. http://www.textbookofbacteriology.net/themicrobialworld/Pseudomonas.html.

AHCC and Cancer

Cowawintaweewat S., S. Manoromana, et al. "Prognostic improvement of patients with advanced liver cancer after active hexose correlated compound (AHCC) treatment." *Asian Pacific Journal of Allergy and Immunology* 24, no. 1 (March 2006): 33–45.

Gao Y et al. "Active hexose correlated compound enhances tumor surveillance through regulating both innate and adaptive immune responses." *Cancer Immunology, Immunotherapy* 55, no. 10 (October 2006): 1258–66.

Ghoneum M. M. Wimbley, et al. "Immunomodulatory and anticancer effects of active hemicelluloses compound (AHCC)." *International Journal of Immunotherapy* X1, no. 1 (1995): 23–8.

Kawaguchi Y. "Effect of AHCC on gastric cancer." *Kiso & Rinsho* (Fundamental Science and the Clinic), Life Science Co., Ltd., (2003): 179–84.

Matsui Y., J. Uhara, et al. "Improved prognosis of postoperative hepatocellular carcinoma patients when treated with functional foods: a prospective cohort study." *Journal of Hepatology* 37, no. 1 (July 2002): 78–86.

Won J.S. "The hematoimmunologic effect of AHCC for Korean patients with various cancers." *Biotherapy* 16, no. 6 (November 2002): 56–4.

World Health Organization. "Cancer." 2011. http://www.who.int/mediacentre/factsheets/fs297/en/.

AHCC and Chemotherapy

Mach C.M., H. Fugii, et al. "Evaluation of active hexose correlated compound hepatic metabolism and potential for drug interactions with chemotherapy agents." *Journal of the Society for Integrative Oncology* 6, no. 3 (Summer 2008): 105–9.

Shigama K., A. Nakaya, et al. "Alleviating effect of active hexose correlated compound (AHCC) for anticancer drug-induced side effects in non-tumor-bearing mice." *Journal of Experimental Therapeutics & Oncology* 8, no. 1 (2009): 43–51.

Sun B., K. Wakame, et al. "The effect of active hexose correlated compound in modulating cytosine arabinoside-induced hair loss and 6-mercaptopurine- and methotrexate-induced liver injury in rodents." *Cancer Epidemiology* 33, no. 3–4 (October 2009): 293–9.

Sun BX and Mukoda T. "Prevention of myelosuppression from chemotherapeutic agents with AHCC." Amino Up Biochemical Laboratory. *AHCC: Research and Commentary* (2008).

Yamazaki M. et al. "Efficacy of AHCC in preventing side effects of chemotherapeutic agents." Teikyo University Graduate Medical Life Sciences Chemistry Department. *AHCC: Research and Commentary* (2009).

Other Chronic Disease

American Diabetes Association. "Diabetes Statistics." 2011. http://www.diabetes.org/diabetes-basics/diabetes-statistics/?utm_source=WWW&utm_medium=DropDownDB&utm_content=Statistics&utm_campaign=CON.

Daddaoua A., E. Martínez-Plata, et al. "Active hexose correlated compound acts as a prebiotic and is anti-inflammatory in rats with hapten-induced colitis." *Journal of Nutrition* 137, no. 5 (May 2007): 1222–8.

Miao G. et al. "Effect of AHCC on progressive destruction of pancreatic islets in the spontaneous type 2 diabetic STD rat." 12th International Symposium of the AHCC Research Association (2004).

Onishi S. et al. "Suppressive effect of AHCC on progression of amyotrophic lateral sclerosis disease in mouse model." 12th International Symposium of the AHCC Research Association (2004).

Wakame K. Protective effects of active hexose correlated compound (AHCC) on the onset of diabetes induced by Streptozotocin in the rat. *Biomedical Research* 20, no. 3 (1999): 145–52.

Using AHCC

Mach C.M., H. Fugii, et al. "Evaluation of active hexose correlated compound hepatic metabolism and potential for drug interactions with chemotherapy agents." *Journal of the Society for Integrative Oncology* 6, no. 3 (Summer 2008): 105–9.

WebMD. "10 Immune System Busters & Boosters." 2009. http://www.webmd.com/cold-and-flu/10-immune-system-bustersboosters.

Glossary

Acetylating: Adding an acyl group to a molecule. An acyl group is composed of several organic compounds, including the neurotransmitter acetylcholine, acetyl-CoA, acetylcysteine, acetaminophen and aspirin (acetylsalicylic acid). In the case of AHCC, the acyl group is added to glucan.

Antibody: A protein on the surface of B cells that is released into the bloodstream or lymph in response to stimulation by an antigen, such as a bacterium or virus and that then neutralizes the antigen.

Antigen: Any substance that is capable of initiating a specific immune response, typically the production of an antibody. Antigens can be bacteria, viruses, fungi, toxins or any other substance that is foreign to the body.

Antioxidants: Molecules that interact with free radicals and stop the chain reaction of damage these radicals can cause. Commonly known antioxidants include vitamins A, C, D and E, beta-carotene, the minerals selenium and zinc and many phytonutrients such as catechins and carotenoids.

Apoptosis: A normal part of the life cycle of the cell in which the cell is programmed to die or "commit suicide." When treating cancer, one goal is to use an approach or substance that induces apoptosis of cancer cells so they die rather than continue to reproduce excessively.

Biological response modifiers (BRMs): Substances that stimulate or restore the ability of the immune system to fight infections and improve its functioning. They may be found in small amounts in the body and can be made synthetically as well. AHCC is a biological response modifier.

Brachytherapy: Also known as seed implantation, brachytherapy is a type of radiation therapy in which radioactive "seeds" are placed inside the cancerous tissue in a way that allows them to attack the cancer cells.

Cell-mediated immunity: Sometimes referred to as Th1 immunity, it activates T cells, such as natural killer cells and macrophages, that attack and destroy antigens.

Chemotherapy: Cancer treatment that involves the use of drugs designed to stop the growth and reproduction of cancer cells by destroying them. In the process, chemotherapy also kills healthy cells. There are dozens of different chemotherapy drugs, with specific drugs prescribed for specific types of cancer. A few of the commonly used chemotherapy drugs include cisplatin, cyclophosphamide, doxorubicin, 5-fluorouracil, methotrexate, paclitaxel and 6-mercaptopurine.

C-reactive protein (CRP): A protein that is produced by the liver, found in the bloodstream and whose level rises with increasing inflammation in the body. AHCC's anti-inflammatory properties can be measured by monitoring its effect on CRP.

Cytokines: Chemical messengers that are secreted by immune cells that signal the type of response to antigens by the immune system. Some of the many different cytokines include interferons, interleukins and tumor necrosis factor, among others.

Cytotoxicity: The ability to produce a toxic (destructive or killing) effect on cells.

Free radicals: Atoms or groups of atoms that have an unpaired number of electrons in their outer shell and which are formed when oxygen interacts with them. Free radicals are highly reactive and can initiate a chain reaction of cell and tissue damage, including damage to DNA and cell membranes that can result in symptoms, disease, aging and death.

Humoral immunity: Also referred to as Th2 immunity, this immune response uses antibodies produced in the B cells to identify antigens that trigger an immune response.

Immune response: How the body recognizes and defends itself against the invasion of bacteria, viruses, fungi and other substances that appear to be foreign and harmful to the body

Immunomodulator: A substance—natural or synthetic—that has the ability to change, suppress or strengthen the immune system.

Immunosenescence: The gradual decline in the integrity of the immune system that occurs as a result of aging. Age-related immunodeficiency makes individuals more susceptible to infectious conditions, including serious diseases.

Interleukins: A type of cytokines that are mainly produced by and act on white blood cells (leukocytes) to signal the type of action required by the immune system.

Leptin: A hormone that has anti-inflammatory properties and that also is involved in fat metabolism and appetite regulation.

Macrophages: A type of white blood cells that "gobble up" and digest cellular debris and disease-causing organisms.

Myelosuppression: A condition in which bone marrow activity is decreased, which results in a reduction in the production of red blood cells, white blood cells and platelets. Myelosuppression is a side effect of chemotherapy and radiation therapy.

Neutropenia: A blood disorder in which there is an abnormally low number of a critical type of white blood cell called a neutrophil. Neutrophils are a primary defense against infections because they destroy bacteria in the blood. Individuals who have neutropenia are at increased risk of contracting a bacterial infection.

Oxidation: The aging and deterioration of cells due to an increase in the activity of oxygen in the body.

Oxidative stress: A situation in which the body is unable to control damage to cells, tissues and organs caused by free radical activity because there is an inadequate amount of antioxidants available. To counteract oxidative stress, the body produces antioxidants and its ability to produce those antioxidants is controlled by genetic makeup and influenced by environmental factors, including diet, lifestyle habits and other factors.

Phagocytosis: A cellular process by which cell membranes "eat" (phago) cells (kytos). In the immune system, phagocytosis is a major mechanism used to remove pathogens and cell waste, such as bacteria, dead tissue cells and mineral particles.

Polysaccharides: Complex carbohydrates, including starches, cellulose and glycogen, that are stored in the liver and metabolized (broken down) into blood sugar and released into the bloodstream as needed. The main polysaccharides in AHCC are acylated alpha-glucans.

SOD: The abbreviation for dismutase, which is an enzyme and powerful antioxidant that is involved in detoxifying activities. SOD removes excessive active oxygen from the body and neutralizes the effects of oxidative stress.

Tumor necrosis factor: A cytokine that is involved in the inflammatory process and which is capable of attacking and destroying cancer cells.

Viral load: A way to measure the severity of a viral infection by counting the amount of virus in the blood or other bodily fluids.

1. *Human Immunology. Yin Z, Fujii H, Walshe T. Effects of AHCC on the frequency of CD4+ and CD8+ T cells producing IFN-γ and/or TNF-α in* **healthy adults**. *2010 Dec; 71(12): 1187-90.* Subjects: 30 healthy adults over the age of 50. Results: AHCC supplementation resulted in the following significant changes compared with base line: (i) The frequency of CD4+ and CD8 + T cells producing IFN-γ alone, TNF-α alone or both increased during AHCC intake. (ii) The frequency of such cells remained high even 30 days after discontinuing AHCC.

2. *Nutrition and Cancer. Terakawa et al. Immunological effect of AHCC in healthy volunteers: a double-blind, placebo-controlled trial. 2008; 60(5): 643-51.* Subjects: 21 **healthy volunteers.** Results: Volunteers supplemented with AHCC had the following significant changes: (i) Greater number of total DCs than at base line and compared with control. (ii) The number of DC1 cells was greater after AHCC intake than at base line and the AHCC group had a tendency to have higher DC1s than control. (iii) DC2s were significantly increased after 4 weeks compared with control. (iv) The allo-stimulatory activity of DC1s was also increased after intake compared with control as measured by the mixed lymphocyte reaction (MLR).

3. *Nutrition Research. Roman BE, Beli E, Duriancik DM, Gardner EM. Short-term supplementation with active hexose correlated compound improves the antibody response to influenza B vaccine. 2013 Jan; 33(1):12–7.* Subjects: 29 healthy adults. Results: AHCC supplementation improved some lymphocyte percentages and influenza B antibody titers over the control. Changes of lymphocyte subpopulations revealed that AHCC supplementation increases CD8 T cells and NK-T cells following vaccination compared with controls.

4. *Journal of Nutritional Science and Vitaminology. Spierings E, Fujii H, Sun B, Walshe T. A Phase I study of the safety of the nutritional supplement AHCC in healthy volunteers. 2007 Dec; 53(6): 536-9.* Subjects: **26 healthy male or female volunteers** between 18 and 61 years of age. Results: Laboratory results and adverse events were reported as follows: (i) Two subjects (7%) dropped out because of nausea and intolerance of the liquid. (ii) Nausea, diarrhea, bloating, headache, fatigue and foot cramps occurred in a total of 6 subjects (20%) but were mild and transient. (iii) There were no laboratory abnormalities.

5. *Japanese Journal of Clinical Oncology. Sumiyoshi et al. Dietary administration of mushroom mycelium extracts in patients with early stage prostate cancers managed expectantly: a phase II study. 2010 Oct; 40(10): 967-72.* Subjects: **74 prostate cancer patients:** 40 prostate patients undergoing expectant management and 34 patients who had already undergone expectant management for 6 months or more. Results: AHCC supplementation resulted in the following changes: (i) Changes in PSA before and after treatment were substantially stable. (ii) In patients for which expectant management had been continued for 6 months or more before the trial, a prolonged PSA doubling time (PSADT) was seen with AHCC administration. Prior to AHCC, 12/31 (39%) of patients had PSADT of 120 months or more, and after 6 months of AHCC administration, 17/31 (55%) had PSADT of 120 months or more. To the lower end, 12/31 (39%) of patients showed a PSADT less than 24 months, and following 6 months of AHCC, this fell to 9/31 (29%). (iii) Anxiety significantly decreased after 6 months of treatment in patients exhibiting strong anxiety before the start of the trial.

6. *Journal of Hepatology. Matsui et al. Improved prognosis of postoperative hepatocellular carcinoma patients when treated with functional foods: a prospective cohort study. 2002 Jul; 37(1): 78-86.* Subjects: 269 consecutive patients with histologically confirmed **liver cancer.** Results: The AHCC group had the following significant differences compared with control group: (i) Longer non-recurrence period. (ii) Increased overall survival rate.

7. *Natural Medicine Journal. Kawaguchi, Y. Improved survival of patients with gastric cancer or colon cancer when treated with AHCC: effect of AHCC on digestive system cancer. 2009 September; 1(1): 1-6.* Subjects: 132 patients diagnosed with **gastric cancer,** 113 patients diagnosed with **colon cancer.** Results: AHCC supplementation resulted in the following difference in survival rate. (i) Improved cumulative 5-year survival rates for patients with gastric cancer (stage IA to stage IIIA) compared with other Japanese institutions. (ii) Improved cumulative 5-year survival rates for patients with colon cancer (stage II to stage IIIA) compared with other Japanese institutions.

8. *Presented at the 40th APA (American Pancreatic Association) November, 2009. Yanagimoto et al. The beneficial effect of AHCC, a health food component, in patients with pancreatic or biliary tract cancer who underwent chemotherapy.* Subjects: 73 patients with **pancreatic or biliary tract cancer** with PS of 0-1 and adequate organ function. Results: AHCC supplementation resulted in the following changes compared with the control group: (i) The hemoglobin (Hb) level after chemotherapy in AHCC group was significantly higher. (ii) The taste alteration after chemotherapy in AHCC group was significantly lower.

9. *Biotherapy. Uno K et al. AHCC improves immunological parameters and performance status of*

patients with solid tumors. 2000 March; 14(3): 303-309. Subjects: **38 cancer patients** and 117 **healthy people**. Results: AHCC supplementation resulted in the following changes compared with the status before intake: (i) Significant improvement in NK cell activity. (ii) Significant improvement in IFN-γ and IL-2 production. (iii) Significant improvement in PS evaluation.

10. International Journal of Clinical Medicine, 2, 588-592 (2011). Parida D, Wakame K, Nomura T. Integrating complimentary and alternative medicine in the form of AHCC in the management of head & neck cancer patients. Subjects: 25 patients of advance state (T3-T4) **head and neck cancer**. Results: AHCC supplementation resulted in the following observations: (i) All patients tolerated AHCC with no added symptoms. (ii) 20 patients reported feeling better and stronger than before at the time of initiation of chemotherapy cycles. (iii) Almost all patients reported better appetites after they started to take AHCC. (iv) In 12 patients who required blood transfusions before chemotherapy cycles, a decrease in the rate of fall of hemoglobin was observed and only 3 patients subsequently required blood transfusions prior to chemotherapy. (v) 22 patients has a reduction of chemotherapy side effects like nausea, vomiting, loose motion/constipation, etc. (vi) Tumors regressed in 11 patients. (vii) 8 patients stabilized.

11. Asian Pacific Journal of Allergy and Immunology. Cowawintaweewat et al. Prognostic improvement of patients with advanced liver cancer after AHCC treatment. 2006 Mar; 24(1): 33-45. Subjects: 44 patients with advanced **liver cancer**. Results: The following results were reported for patients supplemented with AHCC when compared with control group: (i) A significantly prolonged survival. (ii) Quality of life in terms of mental stability, general physical health status and the ability to have normal activities were significantly improved after 3 months of supplementation. (iii) Serum level of albumin and percentage of lymphocytes in blood, were significantly higher. (iv) Slightly increased levels of total IL-12 and neopterin. (v) In the patient who survived more than 24 months, all 6 parameters seemed not to change vitally, showing a good prognosis that correlated with the survival. In addition, the spider nevi (an abnormal collection of blood vessels near the surface of the skin commonly found in liver cancer patients) on this patient's chest disappeared after 3 months of treatment with no new occurrence until 2 years of follow-up. MRI pictures of his liver mass using magnetic resonance imaging from 2002 (the start of treatment) to 2005 showed that there was no change in tumor size and no new lesion appeared.

12. International Journal of Immunotherapy. Ghoneum M. et al. Immunomodulatory and anti-cancer effects of active AHCC. 1995; X1(1) 23-28. Subjects: 11 **cancer patients** with advanced malignancies. Results: Supplementation with AHCC had the following results: (i) A significant decline in TAA occurred in 8 out of the 11 patients with different types of malignancies. (ii) PSA levels in prostate cancer patients and CA 125 levels in ovarian cancer patients decreased as early as 1 to 2 months and reached normal levels within 1 to 4 months. (iii) 9 out of 11 patients demonstrated marked increase in NK activity as early as 2 weeks after treatment. (iv) The percentages of patients with complete remission were as follows: (a) prostatic (66%); (b) ovarian (66%); (c) multiple myeloma (50%); (d) breast, 33% complete remission and 2 partial. (v) In vitro studies showed that AHCC possesses suppressive effects on tumor cell growth.

13. Nutrition and Cancer. Ito, T., et al. Reduction of Adverse Effects by a Mushroom Product, Active Hexose Correlated Compound (AHCC) in Patients With Advanced Cancer During Chemotherapy—The Significance of the Levels of HHV-6 DNA in Saliva as a Surrogate Biomarker During Chemotherapy. 2014 Apr;66(3):377–82. Subjects: 24 patients with cancer. Results: The DNA levels of herpes virus type 6, often found in people with compromised immune systems and thought to be related to chronic fatigue syndrome, were significantly increased after chemotherapy. AHCC significantly decreased the levels of HHV-6 in saliva during chemotherapy, improved QOL scores in the EORTC QLQ-C30 questionnaire and reduced blood and liver toxicity.

14. International Journal of Integrative Medicine. Ishizuka, R., et. al. Review of Cancer Therapy with AHCC* and GCP*; The Long-Term Follow-Up Over 12 Years For stage IV (M1) Cancer of the Lung and the Breast. 2010 July; vol. 2, no. 1. Subjects: 36 patients with stage IB-IV lung cancer and 34 patients with stage IV breast cancer. Results: Compared with the survival rates in American Society of Clinical Oncology reference data, this retrospective study reported the following observations:

- 1-year, 2-year, and 3-year survival rates for stage IV lung cancer increased to 75.0%, 52.1%, and 21.8%, respectively. 4-year survival was 6.2%, and 5-year survival was 0%.
- 41.7% of 36 M1 patients in classes A and B had improved quality of life (QOL).
- Improvement of 1-year to 3-year survival rates and prolongation of median survival time for stage IV lung cancer.
- QOL scores of 35 cases were rated A to C by 77.2% of patients, which contributed to reducing

final hospitalization time.

- Survival terms for breast cancer patients for 1 year, 2 years, 3 years, 4 years, and 5 years were 100%, 84.4%, 68.3%, 36.8%,and 28.1%, respectively.
- Mean survival terms for breast cancer patients were 5 years, 2 months after recurrence and 7 years, 11 months after initial diagnosis.
- Survival terms for breast cancer patients for 3 years, 4 years, and 5 years were 65.6%, 43.8%, and 28.1%, respectively.
- Extension of survival terms was confirmed.
- QOL scores improved 67.7%.

15. *Biotherapy. Jang Seok Won. The hematoimmunologic effect of AHCC for Korean patients with various cancers. 2002 November; 16(6): 560-564.* Subjects: 12 **cancer** patients. Results: AHCC supplementation resulted in the following changes compared with baseline: (i) The ratio of NK cells to total lymphocytes increased from 21.67% before taking AHCC to 26.21% and 26.0% 3 to 6 months after taking AHCC, respectively. (ii) There was no change in white blood cells, hemoglobin, hematocrit and thrombocyte numbers after taking AHCC, even though patients were undergoing radiotherapy or chemotherapy. (iii) No adverse effects were observed.

16. *Presented at 2nd Meeting of the Society for Natural Immunity, May 1994. Ghoneum, M. NK-immuno-modulation by AHCC in 17 cancer patients.* Subjects: 17 **cancer** patients. Results: AHCC supplementation resulted in the following changes: (i) Significant enhancement of NK activity against K562 as early as 2 weeks, two- to threefold increase compared with base line. (ii) Activity was further increased at subsequent time periods up to 6 months post-treatment with AHCC. (iii) NK activation was also detected against Raji cells, but at later stages 1-2 months with two- to ten fold increase compared with base line.

17. *Anti-Cancer Drugs. Turner J, Chaudhary U. Dramatic prostate-specific antigen response with AHCC in metastatic castration-resistant prostate cancer. 2009 Mar; 20(3): 215-216.* Subjects: 1 Caucasian male (66 years old) with **castration-resistant prostate cancer.** Results: The self-administration of AHCC tesulted in a dramatic PSA decrease within 1 month, which continued to control his disease for over 6 months from initial supplementation with AHCC.

18. *International Journal of Integrative Oncology. Matsui, Y, Kamiyama, Y. Retrospective study in breast cancer patients supplemented with AHCC. 2009; Vol. 3 No. 2.* Subjects: 47 patients with various stages of **breast cancer.** Results: Using the National Breast Cancer patient registration as reference data, this retrospective study reported that the AHCC supplementation improved the prognosis in Stage IV as compared to the national counting.

19. *The Medical News (Thailand). Thaiudom S, Piyaniran W, Chutaputthi A. A study of the efficacy of AHCC in the treatment of chronic hepatitis C patients at Phramongkutklao Hospital (2010) 325, 13-16.* Subjects: 39 **chronic hepatitis** C patients. Results: AHCC supplementation resulted in the following changes: (i) Although no significant reduction of HCV RNA levels was noticed in AHCC group patients compared with those of placebo group, subgroup analysis of genotype-3 had a significant HCV RNA decline. (ii) Although the reduction of ALT levels within AHCC group was not significant, a significant difference was found between AHCC and placebo groups. (iii) ALT levels were stable for AHCC group, while ALT levels increased in placebo group, and such difference was initially noted within the first 6 weeks of the study.

20. *Presented at the 18th International Congress on Nutrition and Integrative Medicine (ICNIM), July 2010. Kim J. The Effect of AHCC in non-viral, chronic and abnormal liver function condition: a randomized, double-blind, placebo-control study. (2010).* Subjects: 30 male subjects with **non-viral, chronic and abnormal liver function** conditions. Results: AHCC supplementation resulted in the following changes: 1. 1 g AHCC significantly decreased AST, ALT and γ-GT values. 2. 3 g AHCC significantly decreased AST, ALT and γ-GT values except the 4-week γ-GT. 3. AHCC supplementation had a more dramatic effect on immune cell phenotypes after vaccination of subjects over 60 years old

About the Authors

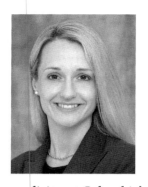

Philippa J. Cheetham, M.D. is a board-certified Urological Surgeon from the United Kingdom (UK). Previously, Dr. Cheetham was an attending physician in Winthrop Urology, PC and was on the medical staff of the Department of Urology at Winthrop-University Hospital. She had also spent several years at Columbia University's Department of Urology focusing on robotic surgery, prostate cryotherapy and integrative medicine at Columbia's Center for Holistic Urology. After graduating with Honors from the University of Bristol Medical School in the UK, she completed a 5-year general surgical training program at The John Radcliffe Hospital University teaching hospital at Oxford University. She was also awarded a prestigious academic research fellowship from the Royal College of Surgeons of England. Dr. Cheetham is the coauthor of the books, *Robotic Prostatectomy for Prostate Cancer—Is It For You?* and *Living a Better Life After Prostate Cancer—A Survivor's Guide to Cryotherapy.* She has also published numerous articles in peer-reviewed journals and presented extensively at prestigious international academic meetings all over the world. Dr. Cheetham is cofounder of The Society of Integrative Urology and is a frequent guest on major national TV and radio shows.